An Offering of Leaves

D0067573

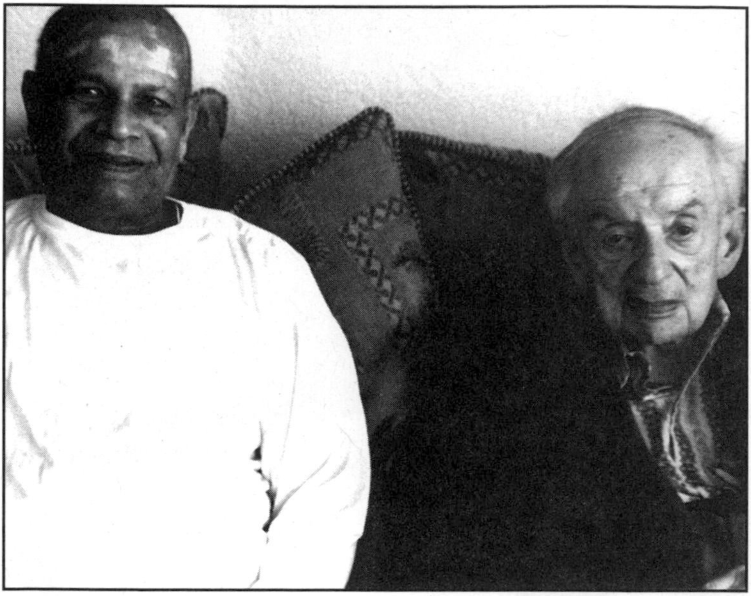

Guruji and my father

An Offering of Leaves

Ruth Lauer-Manenti

Lantern Books • New York
A Division of Booklight Inc.

2009
Lantern Books
128 Second Place
Brooklyn, NY 11231
www.lanternbooks.com

Copyright © 2009 Ruth Lauer-Manenti

All rights reserved. No part of this book may be reproduced, stored in a retrieval system, or transmitted in any form or by any means, electronic, mechanical, photocopying, recording, or otherwise, without the written permission of Lantern Books.

Printed in the United States of America

Library of Congress Cataloging-in-Publication Data

Library of Congress Cataloging-in-Publication Data

An offering of leaves / Ruth Lauer-Manenti.
p. cm.
Collection of teachings given over the last few years at the Jivamukti Yoga School in New York City; the teachings were inspired by monthly essays written by Sharon Gannon.
ISBN-13: 978-1-59056-150-8 (alk. paper)
ISBN-10: 1-59056-150-3 (alk. paper)
1. Religious life—Hinduism. I. Lauer-Manenti, Ruth. II. Gannon, Sharon.
BL1237.36.O55 2009
294.5'432—dc22

2009024003

Lantern Books has elected to print this title on Rolland Enviro, a 100% post-consumer recycled paper, processed chlorine-free. As a result, we have saved the following resources:

12 trees, 332 lbs of solid waste, 31,427 gallons of water,

47,000,000 BTUs of energy, 730 lbs of net greenhouse gases

As part of Lantern Books' commitment to the environment we have joined the Green Press Initiative, a non-profit organization supporting publishers in using fiber that is not sourced from ancient or endangered forests. We hope that you, the reader, will support Lantern and the GPI in our endeavor to preserve the ancient forests and the natural systems on which all life depends. One way is to buy books that cost a little more but make a positive commitment to the environment not only in their words, but in the paper that they are published on. For more information, visit www.greenpressinitiative.org.

green press INITIATIVE

I bow down to the lotus feet of my guru Sri K. Pattabhi Jois

I dedicate this book to my guru Sri K. Pattabhi Jois,
his daughter Saraswati, and grandson Sharath,
to my teachers Sharon Gannon and David Life,
to my teachers Dr. M. A. Jayashree and Prof. M. A. Narasimhan,
and to my parents Stefanie and Lothar Lauer

Acknowledgments

This book is a collection of teachings given over the last few years at the Jivamukti Yoga School in New York City, to the best and most treasured group of students a teacher could ever ask for. The teachings were inspired by monthly essays written by Sharon Gannon. The text has been edited to maintain the directness and immediacy of those talks. Each "talk" can be read on its own, although they are meant to be read in order. This has necessarily meant some repetition.

Rima Rabbath recorded the teachings because she felt they should be documented. Andrea Boyd transcribed them because she loved the teachings, and thought they would make a valuable book. Jessica Kung and Stéphane Dreyfus expertly arranged the Sanskrit for us so we could have the verses in the original alphabet. Katherine Pew showed me how to transition from spoken to written word. Martin Rowe encouraged me, and more importantly, to my great delight, he published the book.

While Andrea is a strong and gifted teacher, she remains a humble student. Only with Andrea by my side could this have been completed. Such devotion and excitement are rare. I thought that if the book made money, it could be given to my friend's orphanage in India, which you can read about in "Children and Animals" and "The Lord Brings Rice."

Additional thanks to: Robert Manenti, Fern Manenti, Michael Lauer, Lisa Shrempp, Professor H. V. Nagaraja Rao, Dr. C. A. Gurudath, Ambika Gurudath, Geshe Michael, Lama Christie, Eddie Stern, Jeffrey Cohen, Ananda Ashram, Mason Tinker, Kimberly Flynn, Lois Conner, Jessica Perry, and Carlos Menjivar.

Contents

Explanation of the Ancient Scriptures Used

The Yoga Sutras

The Yoga Sutras of Master Patanjali are distilled from the teachings on yoga that were contained in the Upanishads, some of which had been composed centuries earlier. *The Yoga Sutras* has four chapters and two hundred sutras. Within the sutras lies the essence or crux of yoga philosophy and practice: How to stop repressing our innate good qualities and allow our true nature to sustain us. The word *sutra* means "thread," or that which holds things together. The sutras are short, as it was expected that they would be memorized and further discussed.

The dates of Master Patanjali vary from 400 BCE to 400 CE. There are various accounts about his birth. One is that he fell (*pat*) from the heavens into drops of ointment (*anjali*) being held in the hands of a childless woman who was praying that she might become pregnant. He fell in the form of a snake with a thousand heads, each head representing a *pandit,* or spiritual teacher. The snake turned into a boy, who became Master Patanjali. It is said that at the time of his birth he caused his mother no pain, such as is also the case in the birth stories of the Buddha and Jesus.

The Bhagavad Gita

A long time ago, perhaps 2100 BCE, there was a warrior named

Arjuna who was destined to go to war with his family, and was despondent. For guidance he went to the lord, Sri Krishna, who was said to be a full incarnation of Vishnu, the god of preservation. The dialogue takes place on a battlefield, which is synonymous with the challenges we face during life and the fight that goes on within one's mind.

Found in the *Bhishma Parva,* the middle section of the *Mahabharata, The Bhagavad Gita,* or "The Song of the Lord," has eighteen chapters. Around the fourth century BCE, Vyasa, the great Vedic poet, used his divine powers to put the story into 700 verses, sometimes called the "700 suns" that dispel the darkness of ignorance. Written in conversational style, the verses are set to meter, and can be sung in temples, caves, villages, and cities, as a form of study, prayer, while working, before eating, waiting for the bus, or anytime. The beauty of the poetry is often compared to the petals of the lotus flower in bloom.

In the verses, the teacher gives the student a way of living that removes suffering and emphasizes kindness, equanimity, karma, renunciation, meditation, and duty. The student is taught to embrace the entire universe, to be easily approachable by others, and to be at home everywhere. The student of yoga is described as a devotee. Thus the guidelines on the path (how to eat, sleep, work, and treat others) are not followed in a wearisome way, but with dedication and love.

When Arjuna's doubts are cleared, his neurosis ends, and ultimately he realizes Sri Krishna's knowledge as his own. Just as the parent wishes for the child to go further in life than he or she, or as the cow wishes for her calf a life free of suffering, the teacher wishes to be excelled by their student. Thus Sri Krishna was fulfilled by Arjuna.

This book is known to be the one book that Mahatma Gandhi kept on his night table.

The Hatha Yoga Pradipika by Yogi Swatmarama was written between the sixth and fifteenth centuries CE. It is for the young or old, educated or uneducated. It defines yoga as a state of mind, where one's individual thoughts have been put aside and the mind is no longer caught in its own pursuits. This is referred to as a mindless or cosmic state of mind, *manomani*. This does not mean that a person becomes thoughtless. On the contrary, one actually sets an example by one's thoughtfulness, as one's mind is freed from thinking only of oneself. By a combined effort of putting the body in different postures (*asanas*), for example, standing on one's head; by holding one's breath or vital air for long periods of time (*pranayama*); by cleaning oneself from the inside (*kriya*), for example, pouring water in one nostril, tilting the head, and letting the water drip out the other nostril; by focusing the eyes at a single point like a candle flame so as to develop concentration (*tratak*); by leading an ethical life (*yama*) occupied in nonviolence (*ahimsa*), with enthusiasm, perseverance, a positive attitude, and the study of scripture (*niyama*)—currents of energy move upwards and the yogi gets this mindless state of mind.

Through these practices (*abhyasa*), and the grace of a guru, or teacher, one is able to drive away the impurities and purify the subtle channels (*nadis*), which are pathways that energy (*shakti*) moves through. As the spinal pathway becomes clear, the yogi hears holy sounds (*nadam*). These sounds awaken previously dormant areas of the brain so that the yogi stops seeing one as two, there are no distinctions between subject and object, and one exists not as a separate individual but as part of a whole, in a reality that is indivisible. Herein we find the basis of Vedanta philosophy, and hundreds of sentences in hundreds of books on the unity in all things. Duality and otherness, us and them, dissolve like salt into water.

The rising of this snakelike energy (*kundalini*) from the base of the spine and ending slightly above one's head transforms the yogi. Negative traits or tendencies within his or her personality disappear permanently and he or she is likened to a lotus flower with one thousand petals. Eventually, the energy moves with such speed that a pin-size hole is pierced at the top of the head and God drips down through it in the form of nectar (*amrit*), thus opening the yogi's third eye at the *ajna chakra*, the point between the eyebrows. One sees the interconnectedness of life, and in that sees God. Absorbed in a greater consciousness, the yogi and anyone in his vicinity is happy. By following the instructions of the guru well and keeping a vegetarian diet, the practitioner frees oneself from fatigue, wipes out diseases, and ultimately skips death.

A Note about the Sanskrit

Most of the teachings that follow begin with a Sanskrit verse—the knowledge of sages, written down in books and preserved as scriptures. The translations are not word-for-word. Rather, they are poetic interpretations I arrived at through the grace and influence of the following masters: Shri Brahmananda Saraswati, I. K. Taimni, Sri Swami Satchidananda, S. Radhakrishnan, Swami Muktibodhananda, Winthrop Sargeant, and Swami Prabhupada.

I found the following sources useful for the Sanskrit *devanagari* script and transliteration:

- *The Yoga Sutras of Patanjali* by Sri Swami Satchidananda
- *The Textbook of Yoga Psychology* by Shri Brahmananda Saraswati

- *Bhagavad Gita, As It Is* by A. C. Bhaktivedanta Prabhupada
- *Hatha Yoga Pradipika* by Dr. M. A. Jayashree
- *Sabda-Dhatumanjari* by Dr. M. A. Jayashree
- Yoga Studies Institute Course Materials by Geshe Michael Roach and Lama Christie McNally

Foreword

David Life

After a full meal, a large raptor soared skyward with the unconsumed portion of his prey. As he rose above the trees blackbirds appeared from many directions. They flew at the raptor, diving and striking. They called him names and swore at him. He flew only with great difficulty because of the heavy corpse and his full stomach. The blackbirds were making his life hell, but he stubbornly continued to cling to his burden. Finally, he had to release his prey in order to flee the annoying blackbirds. As soon as he let go of the prize, the hungry ones followed the corpse down, leaving the raptor alone in the sky. He flew away, having attained freedom from suffering by letting go of greed.

The first humans who questioned the nature of reality looked carefully into their relationships each day with forces of the Cosmos, Nature, and all other Earthly beings for answers to those questions. When they reflected on these experiences, they received insights that were much more profound than the apparently simple nature of daily events would indicate. The planets, stars, winds, waters, plants, mountains, deserts, and especially the nonhuman animals spoke to these attuned individuals. These enlightened predecessors assembled the first wisdom traditions and preserved them in oral teachings—including philosophy, spirituality, magic, dance, music, and the healing arts. The essential tools of these classic teachers were parable, story, scripture, or example, reflection, and insight. These teachings would draw one's attention to the minutiae of daily-life interactions with the natural world around us and how, with careful observation, they reveal the infinity of existence. Communities assembled cultures and histories using various aspects of oral history as a foundation throughout very early times. Succeeding generations of teachers and students of oral traditions allowed cultures, with their myriad distinctive components, to endure.

These early, often foraging and nomadic cultures were transformed when people began to domesticate animals and became interested in agriculture, commerce, and the culture of accumulation. People became more interested in controlling nature (and neighbors) and less interested in communicating with nature (or neighbors). Humans found less time for the old traditions in a blind rush for selfish material gain and the struggle to hold on to their treasures—like the raptor—against an unknown future. When new oral traditions that related to this culture of accumulation appeared at that time, the old wisdom faced extinction from lack of interest. At a crucial moment, the appearance of written language and the scribes who would chip the teachings into stone, or scratch them onto leaves, preserved many of these teachings to this day. Others just disappeared.

Many of us (humans) find ourselves spending too much time in an all-consuming relationship with a sense-numbing virtual entity of the Web, cell phone, GPS, and digital television, and less time appreciating the rich landscape of our first-hand interactions with others. Walk the streets of almost any town or city on this planet and you will likely observe humans talking on cell phones and depriving themselves of the preciousness of the living moment. Look into the windows and you will likely see humans watching plasma screens of their world, and the other beings that they share the world with—living in digital delay. Many humans inhabit a virtual realm populated by beings that don't bite back, talk back, or look back. It is easy to see that this self-centered relationship to the Earth is dysfunctional. The long list of maladies that we see in the world all arise from a deep disconnection from the Earth. These ills point to a future world where nothing is everything, created from a crippled virtual experience.

We may have lost track of the raptors and blackbirds in our own life, of the parables and metaphors of the passing days. Perhaps we all need to be reminded of the imperishable beauty of the interconnected net of existence. These pages could encourage you to become a seeker after experience yourself. Push yourself away from the screen and take a walk in the immortal and real presence of the jewel in each encounter. This book will give you an authentic experience of the clear vision of wholeness reflected in a jewel-like drop of dew on a small leaf, reflecting the infinity of leaves. It will demonstrate a technique for deepening your appreciation of life, so that you would be encouraged to experience it directly, reflect upon it and receive insights, and share your insights with others.

The parables, stories, scriptures, or examples, reflections, and insights that are scribed into this book arise from a modern living oral tradition of teaching. The talks captured on these pages are delivered in a classic style. Ruth Lauer-Manenti's many years of yoga practice, meditation, and vegetarian diet give her an ascetic's eye. Her studies in art, scripture, and philosophy at the feet of masters give her authenticity. The blessed ones know that the gift of life is to experience directly, reflect on those experiences insightfully, and share insights into the nature of reality with others. Ruth accomplishes this sharing, in a living ancient tradition, by relating universal principles revealed in profoundly simple ways in our daily lives. We remember the stories, the verse, the insight, and devotion to truth.

Introduction

In the summer of 2008, I was in Bylakuppe, an area in southern India given over to the settlement of Tibetan refugees. They have built several temples with the help of the Fourteenth Dalai Lama. Geshe Michael Roach spent twenty-three years there learning how to be a good monk. Bylakuppe is not far from Mysore, where Sri K. Pattabhi Jois ("Guruji") and his family live and teach ashtanga yoga. The temples are full of paintings that depict the lessons of the Buddha on how to reach enlightenment.

It was early in the morning and the monks were in the temple chanting. I was sitting on the ground just outside the entrance. The door was open, so I could see everything. Everyone was very generous. An elderly monk came from behind me and slid a piece of cardboard underneath me. He smiled at me, and my cardboard seat felt luxurious. Then, from inside, another monk threw me a round piece of brown bread. Later, yet another monk asked me where I was from.

I, too, tried to be mindful. I had brought nuts instead of sweets as an offering because of the high rate of diabetes among the monks. At the guesthouse, I didn't order more food than I could eat.

Everyone can give something. In that spirit, I offer this book, like a piece of cardboard to sit on.

An Offering of Leaves

पत्रं पुष्पं फलं तोयं यो मे भक्त्या प्रयच्छति ।
तदहं भक्त्युपहृतमश्नामि प्रयतात्मनः ॥२६ ॥

patraṃ puṣpaṃ phalam toyaṃ yo me bhaktyā prayacchati
tad ahaṃ bhakty-upahṛtam aśnāmi prayatātmanaḥ

However humble the offering, be it a leaf, a flower, fruit, or water,
if it is made with love and devotion, I will accept it.

—*THE BHAGAVAD GITA*, CHAPTER NINE, VERSE 26

This verse is from *The Bhagavad Gita,* a conversation between teacher and student. The teacher is the Lord Himself, and the student is any one of us. Because this chapter is right in the middle of the eighteen chapters, it is halfway through the student's journey. We start out in darkness and we end up in light. The journey is a process of purification.

Lord Krishna says that in the middle of your path—not at the beginning, but not at the end—certain secrets will be revealed to you, things that wouldn't make sense beforehand. This is one of those secrets. The secret is to offer something. Krishna says that if your offering comes from love—then you can give even a leaf . . . a flower . . . a fruit . . . or a glass of water. Previously, the student felt that if he wanted to make an offering, it had to be elaborate or expensive.

I read this verse many years ago and liked it. It is poetic and visual. I love fruit. I love flowers. I wanted to memorize the verse and sing it well. I thought I'd ponder this holy verse and it would give my life direction.

Some time passed, I was giving a retreat, and on the last day of the retreat I invited my sister-in-law, Una, and her husband, Isa—who are priests in a Sufi order—to perform a worship ceremony. They came and led this uplifting service: my sister-in-law was dressed in gold, and my brother-in-law wore white and had a long beard, and they had a drummer, who had a regal turban on his head. They read and sung from texts of all different religions. It was wonderful and moving.

As it was getting toward the end, I thought, "Wow, I don't have anything to offer them." I hadn't thought of it.

Whenever guests visit my teacher's school—like a poet comes to read, or a musician comes to play, or a dancer comes to perform—after it's over, my teacher always gets up and gives offerings. Garlands of flowers are made, coconuts are given, money and shawls are presented, and it's a joyous and important part of the event.

I thought, "I've overlooked this. They've come all this way, and I'm empty-handed." Then I remembered that my students had given me some fruit and flowers, which were still pretty fresh, and I contemplated going back to my room to get them. But I was sitting front and center, and thought it would seem rude if I left. I considered asking my assistant Andrea to go get them for me. I looked over at her—I was trying to get her attention—but she was deeply involved in the reverie of the worship, and I didn't want to disturb her and make her run to get something because I'd forgotten it. So I didn't know what to do.

Then this verse came to me. I was sitting on the grass—we were outside, and there were leaves everywhere. And I thought, "Well, I'm going to offer one of these leaves . . . because Lord Krishna has said that if the offering comes from a pure heart, it's acceptable." I was really excited. I picked three leaves and they became precious.

Then the ceremony ended, and I said, "In *The Bhagavad Gita*, Lord Krishna says that if you give an offering out of love, then you can give a leaf. So, in that spirit, I offer you these leaves."

I had these three leaves in my hand. I gave one to the man with the turban, one to my sister-in-law, all in gold, and one to my brother-in-law, all in white. Not one of them acted like they didn't want the leaf, or that the leaf was beneath them. They seemed honored. I gave them the leaves and the verse became alive for me. It wasn't just words on a page anymore. It's a very humble offering, a leaf. When I offered them the leaf, I wasn't puffed up . . . I didn't have a lot of pride about my offering. It was a leaf.

* * *

There was a student, and every time he went to learn teachings from the Buddha he brought gold as an offering. He had so much wealth that he could bring a lot of gold. Then, many years passed, and this man spent all his wealth. He no longer had any gold.

There was one special teaching coming up that he wanted to go to. He thought, "Well, I have nothing to offer. How can I approach the Buddha empty-handed? What to do?" So he decided to go to the Buddha and ask. "Dear Buddha," he said, "I want so much to go to the teachings, but alas I've spent all my wealth. I have nothing to bring to you. What should I do? I don't want to come empty-handed."

The Buddha said, "Oh, your wealth is gone?"

The man said, "Yes."

"Oh! Gold is no longer there? You have no more gold?"

"This is correct," the man replied. "I have no more gold."

"*Oooh!* Your wealth is finished?"

"Yes, it is finished dear Buddha. I have finished with my wealth."

"Oh!" the Buddha added. "Well, you have one garden. Don't you?"

"Yes," the man responded. "I have a garden."

"You grow beautiful things out of that garden, don't you? So many beautiful things grow in your garden?"

"Yes," said the man. "Beautiful, nice things grow in my garden."

"Your dirt is very fertile. So it's a beautiful thing to grow out of that dirt."

"Yes. The dirt is full of nutrients."

"Ah!" the Buddha said. "It's good dirt, is it not?"

"Yes, it's good dirt," the man said.

"Bring me some of that dirt. You have so much of it. Beautiful things grow out of it . . . bring me some of that dirt."

Orthodox and Reformed Temples

अकशात् पतितं तोयं यथा गच्छति सर्गरं ।
सर्व देव नमस्करः केशवं पतिगच्छति ॥

akaśhat patitaṃ toyaṃ yatha gacchati sargaraṃ
sarva deva namaskaraḥ keśavam pratigacchati

Every drop of rain that falls from the sky eventually goes into the ocean. Similarly, any form of worship of any and all gods eventually goes to the same place.

—FROM THE ORAL TRADITION

Dr. Gurudat, my music teacher in India, taught me this verse. As the translation indicates, the verse means that just as every drop of rain eventually reaches the ocean, so there are as many ways to worship as drops of rain, and as many ways to worship as there are people. But everyone's worship eventually reaches the same place.

My parents belong to an Orthodox synagogue in Southern California. They aren't Orthodox, but there's an Orthodox *shul* or religious school very close to where they live. The rabbi there is world-famous. He comes from a family of seven generations of rabbis. My brother, who is Orthodox, said to my parents, "You live ten minutes away from this *shul* where the rabbi is a great and holy man. You should join this synagogue. It's silly to go to a different one." My father said that he didn't like the Orthodox, and he didn't want to go. My brother kept saying, "You ought to try." Finally, my parents checked it out, and found the rabbi irresistible. They've now been going for ten years.

Whenever I visit, I always go with them to the *shul*. I love to hear the rabbi's spiritual talk, called a *drash*. Because the *shul* is Orthodox, there are a lot of rules to be followed. To start with, you're not supposed to drive on the Sabbath, you're supposed to walk. Being that we're not Orthodox, we drive, but park far away, and then walk. Because my mom is in her eighties, that little bit of a walk is a lot for her, so she feels that she's walked to *shul*. When you go inside, you're not supposed to bring anything with you, not even a purse. The idea is that in the house of God, you wouldn't need any things that are in bags. They would be a distraction from your worshipping.

There is a dress code, and women can't be sleeveless, cannot wear slacks, must cover their ankles, and have to wear a hat or something on their head. My mother is always running after me with a doily that she wants to bobby pin to my head. Inside, the women sit with the women, even if you've come with a man. There's a lot of kneeling and standing. It's a long, unabridged service, and when it's over, you get to eat, and you're hungry, because you've been worshipping for so many hours. But you can't just go ahead and eat. You have to wait for the rabbi to bless the food, and inevitably, the rabbi gets held up somewhere. You can't leave without eating. The food is part of the blessing. Also, if you'd like to say "hello" to the rabbi, you can, but only from afar. Women aren't allowed to touch him, although children are. They are exempt from this rule, so they all sit on his lap. There are many other rules, but these are some of the basic ones.

I was once invited by a student of mine to go to *shul* in New York for Yom Kippur. The *shul* was Reformed. People parked right in front of the synagogue and were jingling their car keys after they came inside, carrying backpacks and purses. Women and men were sitting together, even kissing and holding hands. There wasn't too much kneeling and standing; you got to sit back. And everybody went close to the rabbi. The rabbi talked about worshipping God through loving others.

Later, I was thinking about the two *shuls*. Even though they were different, I liked them both. I liked sitting with women only; there was a feeling of sisterhood and solidarity. I liked having to dress appropriately, to show consideration, and hear my mother say, "You look lovely." It made me happy to please her. I enjoyed having to wait for the rabbi to bless the food before eating it, standing there and feeling my stomach growl. I enjoyed not being able to touch the rabbi. And there was something awesome and mysterious about acknowledging him from afar.

In the other *shul*, I liked to sit next to my husband, and I liked being close to the rabbi. I liked that no matter what you looked like, or what you were wearing or carrying, you were accepted and welcomed.

Both places are spaces to be filled with goodness. While the ways of filling those spaces are different, the goodness is the same. In yoga, we are encouraged to worship God, not only in the way that we see God, but to worship God in all forms, and to bow down and respect all the different ways of worship. This is hard because of our conditioning. We're used to a certain way, and if things are done differently, we may be put off, or judgmental. But, if we accept one, and not another, we will continue to see others, and not the One.

Children and Animals

मैत्र्यादिषु बलानि ॥ २३ ॥

maitriyādiṣu balāni

Strength arises out of compassion.

—MASTER PATANJALI'S *YOGA SUTRAS*,
BOOK THREE, SUTRA 23

India is my home away from home—especially Mysore, a medium-sized city in the south. In Mysore, and actually throughout the world, there are children who don't have homes, or they have homes, but they are broken. I have this friend named Shakunthala, who also lives in this town. When she was two, she had polio, and it left her with a leg that doesn't work. On account of that, her family abandoned her, and she was left on the doorstep of an orphanage, where others took care of her. As an adult, she married a man who is also handicapped, and they inherited the house of her husband's father.

Many of the children who live in Mysore who don't have homes have found Shakunthala, and are in her home all the time. She has been teaching them Math, English, writing, sewing, and drawing. It just happened naturally that she formed a school in her home. She is like their mother. In fact, when she had her own child, she said to me, "These children are no different from my own child. I will not make differentiations like that. It will be the same. They should know that they are the same to me." Like that, she is the mother of all these children.

One day, I was with her in her house, and a small girl came in who was very upset. It turned out that one of her classmates had stolen her pencil, and now she had nothing to write with. So another one of the children who had an extra pencil said, "I will give you my extra pencil." The little girl was relieved that she would have something to write with. The other little girl got up to get her pencil. She had a pencil case. She opened the pencil case, and inside were two pencils: one was five inches long, and one was two inches long. These were precious pencils. She gave the one that was bigger to the girl who was so upset, and the girl was happy that she would have something to write with. These children have very little, and so losing a pencil isn't just like, "Oh, I'll just get another." No, they have very few pencils and schoolbooks, and very little paper, clothing, and rice. All of this is very scarce for these children.

Shakunthala's husband, Girish, is a Brahmin, the highest caste in India. But Shakunthala is not a Brahmin: she is of a lower caste; plus, she is handicapped. So, the husband's family pushes her around. They think the marriage should not have occurred. They don't see Shakunthala's kindness. All the time they yell at her and make her do chores. With one bad leg, she's on her hands and knees scrubbing the floor, while they spit on her. In no way does this bother her. She says, "They're only like that because they are indoctrinated. Why should I hold it against them? They do not know. Handicapped people know."

Brahmins wear a string across their torso, underneath their shirt. But it shows around their neck, so everyone knows they are Brahmin. Girish took his string off. He doesn't want people to respect him because he's wearing the string. He wants people to respect him because his wife is taking care of these children. Shakunthala and Girish wish to establish a legitimate orphanage.

This is their dream and ours, too. Proceeds from this book will help facilitate the building of the orphanage, so that it should not remain in the unmanifest state. Anyone who buys this book will be helping these children. Alone, I can only offer so much, but collectively our compassion has no limit.

Maitri is compassion. *Balani* is strength. Master Patanjali tells us that the blessed result of compassion is strength.

* * *

I once went to a fundraiser for Farm Sanctuary, an organization that rescues animals from factory farms. David Life and Sharon Gannon, co-founders of the Jivamukti Yoga method, were receiving the "Compassionate Lifestyle Award." At the event, a movie was shown that depicted the conditions for the animals that live in factory farms. These movies are difficult to watch, but they help reinforce my choice to be vegetarian. In the movie, you see animals in cages so small that they can't switch directions. Their feet are chained together, or they're chained to the cage; they're filthy, and birds get their beaks cut off, and then they're dragged from here to there. Eventually they're slaughtered.

I was watching the movie as I ate my seven-course vegan meal, which included lasagna and chocolate cake. I was thinking how strange it is that people think they will get strength from eating animals. I was thinking that it's actually in *not* eating animals that the strength derives. Whether it's orphans or animals, love is what makes us strong. Compassion is what will empower us.

Preserving the Lineage

हठविद्यां हि मत्स्येन्द्रगोरक्षाद्या विजानते ।
स्वात्मारामोऽथवा योगी जानीते तत्प्रसादतः ॥ ४ ॥

haṭhavidyām hi matseyendraghorakṣādyā vijānate
svātmārāmo'thavā yogī jānīte tatprasādataḥ

Yogi Matseyendranath had the knowledge of hatha yoga, gave it to Gorakhnath and others, who then gave it to Yogi Swatmarama, who learned it.

—*THE HATHA YOGA PRADIPIKA*,
CHAPTER ONE, VERSE 4

Once upon a time, a student held the teacher's hand and something of this vast and supreme knowledge was transferred. This transference of knowledge is endless.

The Hatha Yoga Pradipika is for the serious yoga student. My teacher says this book is mandatory. As with any subject, there are certain books that one should know well. When we embark on the study of any scripture, it should cause us to bow our heads and to hope that something will sink in. We should feel blessed to be reading such a special book.

At the beginning of the book, the author, Yogi Swatmarama, says that this knowledge came to him from his teacher Gorakhnath, and it came to Gorakhnath from his teacher Matseyendranath, and the knowledge goes all the way back to the original teacher, Shiva. Yogi Swatmarama is acknowledging that, through the grace of others, he has this knowledge to give. He did not come up with this. It goes all the way back to the Lord. We find this in Master Patanjali's *Yoga Sutras* as well, with Ishwara as the teacher of all teachers. This is the lineage.

When you're in a yoga class and the teacher says, "Straighten your arm," and you get a tug, that teacher has also been in a yoga class, where their teacher said, "Straighten your arm," and they got a tug. When the teacher is talking about kindness, and you feel nourished by their words, something inside of you is stirred and something that was sleeping awakens. This is because that teacher also had a teacher who spoke about kindness and woke them up. You reach a point where you feel incredible gratitude toward your teacher and you want to be with them, and bring flowers, coffee, candy, and gold.

My friend John Brady works to save ancient, holy books such as *The Hatha Yoga Pradipika,* particularly those volumes in India that are rotting and being eaten by ants. My Sanskrit teacher in India knows where all these books are, and since John was going to India, I thought they should meet.

"I don't know her last name," I said to John, "because everyone just calls her Jayashree. I don't know the name of the road that she lives on, and I'm not sure about the house number, and I don't have her phone number or email. But, if you're standing right in front of the Jagan Mohan Palace, make a left turn and go down a block. You'll get to a man that sells cucumbers. Once you get there, turn right, and go down that road, and you'll get to a pink house with yellow trim. When you get there, turn left, and go down that road, and after awhile you'll get to this big old tree that's a shrine, where they've tied string around it and tucked pictures of holy people in the crevices. When you get to that tree, turn left at the next road, and you'll see a house with motorcycles parked in front. Go in that house, walk through it, and go out the back door to a little alley. Go through the alley, and it's the third house on the right."

John looked a bit overwhelmed and I got the sense that he might not go. I told him, "You've got to. Promise me you'll go." So he went and found the precious teacher. Through their meeting, Jayashree was able to introduce him to the great librarians of India, and he received access to ancient yogic texts. John has employed Tibetan refugees to digitize the texts so that they can be electronically preserved. All because he looked for the cucumber man and the pink house. . . .

This is what keeps the tradition healthy and alive. All the links that keep a student close to their teacher and a book intact become a chain that when unbroken is called a lineage. Yogi Swatmarama is saying that you are being entrusted with a whole lineage, and if you listen well, knowledge survives.

Pickled Peppers

ते लि य ले रु राम भक्ति मर्ग ई ल ल ई नन् तत् अः ॥

te li ya le ru raama bhakti marga ī la la ī nan tat aḥ

How can I be a better devotee? How can I open my heart? Let me cry not for my own disappointments, but because life is large and touching.

—COMPOSED BY TYAAGARAJA (1767–1847), THE CRYING SAINT WHO LONGED FOR THE LORD

My husband and I have a cabin in upstate New York. Near the cabin is a fantastic farm stand that's been around for generations. The men do the farming, their wives sell the produce, and the children help. For instance, if you buy a big watermelon, one of the kids will carry it to your car for you. The stand is outdoors, but partially covered, and the vendors write everything down on a paper bag—mushrooms $1, flowers $4—and then they add the amount up in their heads.

One time I was there, I met a man in his seventies. He had a cloth bag and I noticed he was buying about thirty bell peppers and I thought he must have a plan, a recipe. So I asked him what he was going to do with so many bell peppers and he replied, "I'm going to pickle them."

And I said, "Oh."

He said, "Yes, you put them in a jar, with salt and vinegar, then you can eat them all through the winter. They're very good. When my wife was alive, we used to pickle everything. We would pickle beets, carrots, and string beans. But now I just pickle the peppers." And when he said that to me, I thought I was going to cry. But I pulled myself together, wished him a good day, and said it was nice to meet him.

I went home and told my husband about this man and started to cry—but not over my own disappointments. This was a different kind of crying. It wasn't about something in my personal life. I was just so touched by this man's life that I cried. There was nothing vain or superficial about it. The loss of his wife from a marriage of many years of pickling vegetables together cut right through me.

Handmade Perfection

पूर्णमदः पूर्णमिदं पूर्णात् पूर्णमुदच्यते ।
पूर्णस्य पूर्णमादाय पूर्णमेवावशिष्यते ॥

pūrṇam adaḥ pūrṇam idaṃ pūrṇāt pūrṇam udacyate
pūrṇasya pūrṇam ādāya pūrṇam evāvaśiṣyate

Purna is full, whole, intact, complete, perfect, golden, fat with goodness, fat with joy, robust. No matter what you give, what you're left with is full, and what you give is full. It is perfect, it is whole, it is complete, it is fat.

—AN INVOCATION FROM THE *ISHA UPANISHAD*

During the Depression, there was a group of women who made quilts, called Gee's Bend. They were part of a black community in Alabama who wanted to keep their children warm and well fed, so they made and sold quilts. They were very poor, so they used inexpensive materials. Then, a few years back, these quilts were displayed in a museum. There was a movie that went along with the exhibit, and some of the women who had made these quilts were interviewed. They were in their eighties at that point in time.

In the movie, one woman explained that the quilts were made by sewing squares together. One time, she needed twelve squares for a quilt. She sewed eleven and then, when she had one more to sew, she realized she didn't have enough fabric. She had little money and couldn't just go and buy more. She wondered, "How will I finish my quilt?" Then she found an old pair of trousers that her children had outgrown, and cut them so they were flat, and made the final square out of them.

When you look at these quilts, you would never think that because one square is different from the rest, these quilts aren't perfect. They're complete. Nothing is missing. They're stunning. All the hardship, resourcefulness, and love that is in these women is woven into these quilts. They're handmade. They reflect depth of character and depth of life.

I think sometimes we have a conditioned idea of what perfect is. Perfect would be like every square being the same, or having exactly the right amount of fabric. But in this case, the perfection of these quilts, just like our perfection, is large enough to contain imperfections, irregularity, or surprise. It's not that the woman thought beforehand, "I'll make eleven squares one way and then I'll make the twelfth out of my child's trousers."

It's inspiration that makes the quilt perfect, not the pattern or the fabric. Making mistakes is a part of life. It keeps us humble and resourceful, and therein lies our perfection—just like the quilts.

Shakunthala's Birthday

अशक्यतत्त्वबोधानां मूढानामपि संमतम् ।
प्रोक्तं गोरक्षनाथेन नादोपासनमुच्यते ॥ ६५ ॥

aśakyatattvabodhānāṃ mūḍhānāmapi saṃmatam
proktaṃ gorakaṣanāthena nadopāsanamucyate

The sound of God can be heard even by the unlearned.

—*THE HATHA YOGA PRADIPIKA,*
CHAPTER FOUR, VERSE 65

Nadam is the sound of God, which can be heard by all when the mind is still.

Sometimes if you're at the right place at the right time, you may hear something that causes your own individual mind to stop. All of your thoughts dissolve, and all that is left is beyond.

I have a dear friend in India named Shakunthala. Shakunthala means "feather of a peacock." In my mind, she has a very hard life, because she has polio. Her family saw her as flawed and a financial hindrance, and so abandoned her, and she went from one orphanage to the next.

One year I was in India, Shakunthala's birthday was coming up, and I was thinking I'd like to do something special for her—maybe take her out to eat, or go to the spa up on the hillside. I asked her if she had plans for her birthday. She said, "Yes" and lit up. "I've been saving money all year and I have enough to buy rice and dhal to cook and take to the orphanage nearby in Mysore." So, on her birthday, she was going to see these children to give them love, affection, and food.

I'm listening to her and thinking, "Gosh. I was going to take her to the spa or to dinner." As I was standing there, I could feel the shift of energy, as I was being lifted out of ordinary dullness. I recognized that I was standing in the presence of real wisdom. This ascension of energy is a fundamental principle of yoga, and what I heard awakened my goodness. I will always remember how I felt when I heard Shakunthala say what she was doing on her birthday. I know that having explored what that meant to me has completely changed what I do on my birthday. They say that what you do on your birthday sets the tone for the rest of the year.

Take Your Co-Workers to Lunch

विधिहीनमसृष्टान्नं मन्त्रहीनमदक्षिणम्।
श्रद्धाविरहितं यज्ञं तामसं परिचक्षते ॥१३॥

vidhi-hīnam asṛṣṭānnaṃ mantra-hīnam adakṣiṇam
śraddhā-virahitaṃ yajñaṃ tāmasaṃ paricakṣate

Work without spiritual direction, offerings of food, sacred songs, or donations, is empty of faith and tamasic. It makes one dull and puny.

—*THE BHAGAVAD GITA*,
CHAPTER SEVENTEEN, VERSE 13

This verse from *The Bhagavad Gita*, like many throughout the *Gita*, concerns work. Lord Krishna says that everybody must work, and that if the main reason we work is not to benefit society, but to make money simply to buy things, then things control us. So desire for things should not be the number one reason we work.

Lord Krishna tells us that work should be done in the name of service. We all have gifts. We can find a way to be generous and use our gifts through our work. Our work need not be something separate from our *sadhana* or spiritual practice.

Yoga is a practice where we try to integrate all the different aspects of our being, so that every moment of our life is spiritual. So, it's not like you just turn that off when you go to work. If you're a Buddhist, you're a Buddhist at work. If you're a yogi, you're a yogi at work. Otherwise your work will be insincere.

You shouldn't lie when you're at work. One time—well, I'm sure it's been more than one time—but one time in particular, I remember giving the dates of my vacation. I told my boss that I was going to India for six weeks. In fact, I was going on a ten-day meditation retreat, then to Maine for a week, and then to India. However, I made it sound as if I was going to be in India the whole time. So I lied about my vacation. Ordinarily, we may not see this as problematic, but actually to lie like that causes a lot of agitation and makes us very small.

In the verse, Lord Krishna says that if there are no offerings of food, our work will be dull, tamasic. We used to have staff meetings at the yoga center, and Carlos, the manager, would bring big, red, globe grapes. He'd wash them and put them in a bowl. It was nice that he took the time to do this, and it brought everyone together to eat among the co-workers. Carlos paid for the fruits—it was his offering.

I once had a job in a print shop. When it was lunchtime, the owner brought out menus from all the restaurants in the area. The shop was on Canal Street in Manhattan, and there were many Vietnamese, Chinese, Italian, and other restaurants of all kinds. Every day, the owners bought lunch for the employees. They made that offering. We sat around a big table and had lunch together. It was civilized and old-fashioned in a wonderful way. If you have an opportunity to buy a co-worker lunch, take it. Feeding each other is one of the most human ways we have of expressing love. If you have people who work for you, take them out to eat once in a while. It's very important. Make that gesture.

Lord Krishna says that you should contribute to the workplace. For instance, if the place where you work has a fundraiser, donate to the fundraiser, be supportive. If someone where you work is sick, and they take up a collection, contribute. If your colleagues are buying a birthday present for the boss, chip in, so you're part of that birthday present. Anything where there is money being collected for a good cause, chip in. Watch out for that puny monster that says, "Don't give."

There should be song in our work. My husband Robert works at St. Vincent's, which is a Catholic hospital. They play the Lord's Prayer over the intercom at eight o'clock every morning. He says it's really nice—everyone just takes a moment. It's an old, crackling recording of a nun from the 1930s. It's a precious tradition that they have. Lord Krishna is saying that you should look for ways to bring song into your work. Even if you were just singing quietly to yourself, you wouldn't be working begrudgingly; there would be this cheer that you would have to your work.

We may think we're successful if we're making lots of money, but our success can be much greater if these things—truthfulness, offering food, charity, and song—are a part of our work.

Yogis want to work for God. We want to be useful. We have a trust that God will work through us, and we will thereby benefit society. We'll be receptive and egoless enough that some magic will work through us. We want to be Divine workers.

Knitting Blankets

क्रमान्यत्वं परिणटामान्यत्वे हेतुः ॥ १५ ॥

kramānyatvaṃ pariṇaṭāmānyatve hetuḥ

The order of things causes how things turn out.

—MASTER PATANJALI'S *YOGA SUTRAS*,
BOOK THREE, SUTRA 15

Krama is the order of things. We see it in the seasons. *Anyatvam* is differences or variety. We see it in the flowers. *Parinama* is change. We see it in our lives, as we go from one thing to the next. Master Patanjali is saying that the order of things determines how we change and where we end up.

In India, a typical example of this sutra would be: you take earth, mix it with water, end up with clay, roll it out, pick out the pebbles, make it smooth, form a bowl, bake the bowl, paint it, pour some water in the bowl, take two lotus flowers and put them in the water, and place it on the altar in front of the picture of your guru. The bowl didn't appear out of nowhere, it came from the earth.

I went to the Museum of Art and Design in New York City to see a show about the relationship between crafts and fine arts. In the art world, there is a hierarchy. Painting and sculpture are at the top, while basket weaving and ceramics are closer to the bottom. That hierarchy has been questioned over time and sometimes thought to be false.

I liked the show very much, but was getting tired. There was one last piece to see. It was a table with numerous skeins of yarn and knitting needles. Attached to the needles were squares of yarn already knitted. On the table was a sign explaining that the knitted squares would be used for blankets for wounded U.S. soldiers coming back from Iraq and Afghanistan. If they're wounded so much that they cannot make the trip all the way back to the U.S., the blankets are sent to a hospital in Germany where there are thousands of soldiers.

The hospital is located in a very cold part of the country, and even though I find it hard to believe, there is a shortage of blankets for these soldiers. A woman started a project where people come together and knit squares, which are then assembled into blankets. Several thousand blankets have been made and sent to this hospital so that each soldier gets his own blanket. I read the sign and looked at the knitted squares and thought, "I know how to knit! I can knit!"

I'd only learned a few months previously because my dear friend Barbara had had a baby, and wanted me to be the godmother. To initiate my becoming the godmother, I thought I should learn to knit, so I could make the baby a blanket. Fern, my husband's mother-in-law, is eighty-five years old, and has been knitting since she was five. I asked her to teach me. She gave me lessons, and we became good friends. She told me many stories about her life. When I was done with the blanket, she said, "It needs a little something. I will crochet rosettes around the borders of the blanket." So she did, and when people visit Barbara to see her baby, they ask to see the blanket.

I sat down in that museum and I knitted until it closed. Normally I do everything slowly, but I was knitting quickly—not out of aggression, but out of inspiration. That inspiration was fuel. I signed up to knit a square every month. I felt connected to the soldiers who are wounded, cold, and abroad, and thought about this while I was knitting. I also felt connected to my fellow knitters—men and women. We weren't speaking because we were busy knitting and our silence created a good atmosphere between these so-called strangers and me.

Because I was able to make something for someone I don't know—who's cold, wounded, and not with his family—I believe my sense of where "me" ends and "you" begins changed. When I learned how to knit, I didn't know that I would be able to knit a blanket for a soldier. I was learning how to knit for a baby. But, in retrospect, I can see that what I had learned back then, the Lord could now use. I had this skill to pull out of my pocket.

Let's say you learn French, and then someone in the subway has a panic attack and only speaks French, and no one else in the car speaks French but you. Then you'll know why you learned French. So with a sequence of events, no effort is ever lost. If you're going to make the journey, you have to believe in the journey. You have to know that each thing that you learn is going to be used. Knitting is a beautiful activity . . . no longer at the bottom of the hierarchy.

Seeing Ourselves

लोकः समस्तः सुखिनो भवन्तुः

lokaḥ samastaḥ sukhino bhavantuḥ

May all beings everywhere be happy and free.
May I offer my life to all beings everywhere.

—A MANTRA

I've been going to India for many years and I always go to Mysore. I've made friends with some of the Indian people in this town, particularly Shakunthala. Shakunthala takes care of children in a very informal way, they follow her home and then she feeds and teaches them. Over the years, I've come to know some of these children. Sometimes I'll ask Shakunthala about a specific child, and she'll tell me he or she needs medicine, food, money for school, books, clothes, or a Braille watch. There's always something they need. I'll ask about the cost and she'll tell me it's anything from two dollars to a hundred dollars, and I'll say, "I'll pay for it." When I get home and look at my bank statement, I see that I have converted the currency incorrectly, not in my favor but always on their behalf. So, I've seen myself give to these children over and over again.

When my cat Nellie got very sick, she spent two weeks in the hospital, and died. My husband and I were hit hard, not only by the death, but also by the bill, which was equivalent to what I earn in a year. We were shocked and we weren't sure how we were going to pay it. Every day, they would send a bill. I knew they were bills because they said "Billing Department" on the upper left-hand corner of the envelope. When they came, I put them off to the side, and started a pile.

A month passed. Then, one day, I opened all fifteen of them. Eleven were identical, but the twelfth showed that a significant portion of the bill had been paid. Then I opened up the next and it indicated another significant amount had been settled. Then I opened up the last, which showed we had no balance due. I asked my husband, "Did you pay the bill at the animal hospital?"

"No," he replied.

I said, "Well, come and look at this."

So he did. We figured out that somebody must have paid it, and I started crying. My husband, Robert, said, "We'll call the hospital and find out who paid it, and pay them back." The hospital told us they were under strict instructions not to tell us who had paid. Then Robert said, "Well, look, if they wish to remain anonymous, then let's just leave it. Let's honor their wish. It's a good thing." So we left it.

I see myself as a person who gives, because I've given to these children year after year. I've seen myself in many ways over my life, both giving and not giving. You see yourself do everything that you do, and it leaves an imprint, a *samskara*. Then that imprint is projected out into the world. If I see myself as someone who gives, then I will live in a world where I see others in that same way. That's how we create our world.

What would be the projection of the action of eating meat? If we eat a slaughtered animal, we eat a carcass. The animal is dead when we eat it, it's been killed violently: an animal whose spirit has been dismissed, whose life has not been encouraged. If we see ourselves eating that, then how will we see our world? What will our projection be? What are we creating from what we eat? I don't think we like to ask ourselves these questions too often. Al Gore had a great title for his film on global warming, *An Inconvenient Truth.* Yoga has a lot of inconvenient truths. But, if you want to make the world better, then these inconvenient truths need to be embraced.

Bending the Rules

अत्याहारः प्रयासश्च प्रजल्पो नियमाग्रहः ।
जनसङ्गश्च लौल्यं च षड्भिर्योगो विनश्यति ॥ १५ ॥

atyāhāraḥ prayāsaśca prajalpo niyamagrahaḥ
janasaṅgaśca laulyam ca ṣaḍbhiryogo vinaśyati

These are guidelines to help the yogi on their journey to enlightenment. Following an inner voice, the yogi travels to the heart of oneself. During this process, friendliness, silence, and love grow. One becomes sensitive to all of life, and the whole world becomes one's family. This journey is blocked by keeping the stomach overfull, straining one's self, overworking physically or mentally, constantly blabbering, following rules blindly and rigidly, watching television, and lacking order, discipline, and routine in one's life. These obstacles, or distractions, should be discarded, so that one's energy can be used for spiritual purposes.

—*THE HATHA YOGA PRADIPIKA*, CHAPTER ONE, VERSE 15

We are taking a journey, and that journey is taking us deep inside ourselves. We come to know ourselves. Oh, happy day, when we realize our true nature! Not to just feel ourselves as gross, selfish, irritable beings, but to go beyond, to know our spirit, and not just our personalities. We are not the first to make this journey. So many human beings, from different times and places have also made this journey, and guidelines have been written by them to help us. They are very straightforward.

If you eat, and you make yourself full, and then you keep eating, you will have a stomachache and need a nap. Then, if you take a yoga class, you feel a little better. Some time passes and you overexert yourself, you have a problem, and you spend hours worrying about it. Again you're in a funk, then you go take a yoga class and feel better. You have some relief from all that mental strain. Time passes and you're blabbering and it's making you agitated, then you go take a yoga class, and again feel better. Afterwards, you go home and eat too much and watch television, and go to sleep. In the morning, you don't feel so good, and you go take a yoga class, and feel better.

This segment of *The Hatha Yoga Pradipika* explains that if your lifestyle is like this, then your yoga practice might help you feel better; but if you continue doing things that make you feel worse, you won't be going very far on your journey. You can see how you won't go far that way. This is why rules are helpful. But even rules have their exceptions.

I want to give an example about not adhering to rules rigidly. I was in California where my parents live and my guru, Sri K. Pattabhi Jois, was visiting that area. I had the idea that I would introduce my parents to my guru and so I arranged it. In India, there is this rule that before you go into most places, you take your shoes off. It's a strict rule, especially before you go into a place where there's a holy person. You always leave your shoes outside.

When we were in the car driving to where Guruji was staying, I realized my father would have to take his shoes off. He is very old and has really sore feet, so I knew this would be difficult for him. I was thinking, I can't ask him to take off his shoes. He's already making a huge effort by getting dressed and going out of the house to meet Guruji. But the rule is a tradition. It's got hundreds of years behind it. I've never seen shoes in Guruji's household, so I didn't know what to do.

When we arrived at the house, I said to my parents, "Wait in the car and I'll tell Guruji that we're here, and come back to get you." I knocked on the door, and Guruji's grandson Sharath came to the door. I said, "We're here, but my dad is very old and he has very sore feet. It would be hard for him to take off his shoes. Is it going to be a problem?" Guruji overheard this and wanted to know what was going on, so I went in and told him. Guruji said, "No problem, no problem. Let him come. Let him come," with this great big smile on his face.

Guruji could see the goodness behind my intention, that I was looking out for my father, who's old and who would have been embarrassed to be slow in taking off his shoes. At the same time I was being respectful of his tradition, not dismissing it. I was trying to be a good student and a good daughter. Guruji could see that. And so in this case we did not adhere to that rule. It is important to follow rules—they are good; they help keep order in our life. But it's important to break them at times.

Roderick and the Infinite

स्थिरसुखमासनम् ॥ ४६ ॥

sthira sukham āsanaṃ

Asana is that which is steady and joyful. By various postures, imbalance and tension in the body are released.

—MASTER PATANJALI'S *YOGA SUTRAS*, BOOK TWO SUTRA 46

प्रयत्नशैथिल्यानन्तसमापत्तिभ्याम् ॥ ४७ ॥

prayatna śaithilyānanta samāpattibhyāṃ

Asana is effort turning into balance turning into stillness turning into revelation.

—SUTRA 47

ततो द्वन्द्वानभिघातः ॥ ४८ ॥

tato dvandvānabhighātaḥ

Then, one is no longer disturbed by opposites.

—SUTRA 48

These are the three sutras on *asana*. Master Patanjali tells us that *asana* is posture that is steady and joyful. He explains that it is steady because the practitioner applies effort, but at the same time is relaxed. There's a time in practicing an *asana* where we find poise; balance is there. It is joyful because the mind is focused on the infinite, not on something petty. Then the *asana* practice is correct. Master Patanjali says that, as a result of postures that are steady and joyful, one is no longer afflicted by opposites: pain and pleasure, joy and sorrow, hot and cold no longer afflict the yogi.

Through correct practice of *asana,* mental and physical tension goes, and what we're left with is goodness, and we feel relieved. We find something that was always there, that no one else had to tell us about. It is like having a huge bank account, but not knowing about it. You think you're poor, and the banker is wondering why you never come and get your money.

Some people believe that the yogi is cool and indifferent, unaffected by the ups and downs of the world. That is not so. Through the practice, one's sensitivity increases, and the practitioner becomes less in denial of the pain and suffering that goes on in the world, and more affected. But one is not afflicted, because one is anchored by goodness. What else is going to anchor you?

I have a dear yoga student named Roderick. He lives in New York City, and has hair down to his knees. One time, he broke his back and had to go to the doctor in New Jersey. A friend drove him, so he wouldn't have to take public transportation. Now, New Jersey's not far from New York City: India's far! Roderick said that the journey was very painful. It was hard for him to be in a car and go all the way to New Jersey. Then he thought of all the people who can't just go wherever they want because they are in pain. Like my father always wants to go to Vienna, because that's where he grew up, but he's so old it's hard for him just to walk from the kitchen to the dining room. How would he go all the way to Vienna?

So, Roderick realized that for his whole life he had taken his agility and mobility for granted. Now, just going to New Jersey was difficult. Within this realization, he felt a vastness. This is what Patanjali is saying: Focus on the infinite. Roderick didn't feel, "Oh, my back, my injury, my life has been interrupted." Instead, he felt, "Oh, I now understand how it feels to be in pain, and what it's like to have your life dictated by what you can and can't do because of pain." This compassion grew in him. As a result of his accident, he became less self-absorbed. Thus he was affected, not afflicted.

Wealth on an Empty Kitchen Table

A rich merchant was preparing to go on a business tour. A thief, eager to rob the rich man came to him, dressed in fine clothes, and pretending to be a merchant himself, said, "I also have to travel the same route. It is not safe to venture forth alone when one is carrying money. Let us make the journey together." It was agreed.

In the morning before starting from the inn, the merchant would take out all his money, count it carefully, and put it back into his pocket. He did this quite openly, while the thief was watching him and planning to steal the money that very night. After a tiring day, they settled down to rest 'til sunrise and soon the merchant was fast asleep. The thief had kept awake. He got up from bed and searched his companion's luggage, his bedding, and his person. The merchant never as much opened his eyes, but went on snoring peacefully. Try as he might, the thief failed to discover even a single farthing.

This went on day after day. Every morning, the merchant counted his money, making the thief's mouth water, but at night, no money was to be found. Finally, in his despair, the thief decided to question the merchant.

"Friend," he said, "I must make a confession. I was deceiving you. I really sought your company to get hold of your money. Every night I tried my hardest, but all my efforts to lay my hands on your treasure proved futile, although I searched very thoroughly. Do, please tell me by what magic you kept your money hidden from me."

"It is quite simple," said the merchant, laughing heartily. "From the beginning, I suspected your evil intentions, yet I was quite free from anxiety, be-

cause I knew that you could never guess my hiding place. Every night, the money was lying safely, under your own pillow. I was sure that this was the one place you would never search, and so I was able to sleep most peacefully."

"God is within everyone," comments Mataji. "But man goes out in search of him."

—ANANDAMAYI MA

This is the teaching we get repeatedly from the masters of yoga—that we look for happiness and God outside, when God is inside.

My husband and I borrowed a book from our neighbor. A year went by and we still had the book. Then I saw my husband leaving the house with the book, and I said, "Oh, are you returning that book?"

He said, "Yes, Mary is outside."

I said, "Don't you think we should give her something else besides just the book, since we've had it for a whole year?"

"Like what?" he asked.

On our kitchen table was a ceramic vase that's over a hundred years old, with paintings on it of flowers and birds—a most beautiful vase. In it was a bouquet of flowers that I'd been admiring, made up of several bouquets that students had given me. I said to my husband, "Why don't you take that vase, with those flowers in it?"

"OK," he said. He took both and went to return the book to Mary.

After he left, I turned and looked at the kitchen table, where the flowers and vase had been. In that moment, when I saw that empty space, I could feel my spirit, and I felt happy. The wealth was inside of me, and not on the kitchen table.

So Many Broken Hearts

shalom, shalom, shalom

peace, peace, peace.

Last year on Yom Kippur I went to synagogue. As I was beginning to back into a parking spot, this man drove in from behind. We had a big argument. I was all riled up and I walked into the *shul.* The minute I entered, the rabbi was saying, "Love God by loving others." Immediately, I felt reoriented.

Yom Kippur is a beautiful holiday where you think so deeply that you don't eat, because that's said to be a distraction. You reflect on the past year, how you may have strayed away from all that is good and sacred within you, and where you've gone down the wrong road. Just in acknowledging your wrong roads, you find yourself back on track. This is the essence of this holiday. Because it is so easy to go down the wrong road, there should be at least once a year, if not once a day, an opportunity to stop eating and take inventory.

I always miss my mom and dad on Yom Kippur. I think holidays are like that. Even if you don't have good memories of them, family always comes up. My parents are out in California, and I hadn't arranged to see them for Yom Kippur. So, I was glad when a student of mine gave me a ticket to *shul* in New York, because it's hard to get a ticket for Yom Kippur. Jews who don't go to synagogue all year, do so on Yom Kippur, and the rabbi always says, "Where have you been all year?"

There are a lot of prayers for peace sung on this day. Then there is a memorial ceremony, where you remember a relative or loved one who has passed away. Normally, you give the person's name to the rabbi before the service and then, at a certain point, the rabbi reads them off. My father would always complain that he couldn't hear the names, because the rabbi read them with such speed. They're read quickly because there are many of them.

But this rabbi did something I've never experienced before. He passed a microphone around the congregation and if you had lost someone, you would say, "I want to remember my father, Herman Rothenberg." Or, "I want to honor Minnie Moschowitz." People were encouraged to speak so some healing could occur. This went on for two hours.

So many people had lost people. Somebody said, "My father passed away, he was 102. He had a good life and he died smiling in his sleep." A young woman said, "I want to remember my husband." She could barely get the words out. One lady had left her family in Scotland and moved to New York to be an artist. She spoke of her grandmother who wrote her letters every week telling her about the family. The grandmother loved cooking and would give lengthy descriptions of the different dishes that she had made for family Sunday dinner, and what she might make for next Sunday. The lady was so sad she wouldn't be getting these letters anymore. She wouldn't know what they were eating. Another lady worked with a man who sang to children in hospitals. She said that while he sang, the monitors showed that the blood pressure and heart rate of the patients would normalize; he was like magic. She said that he had died tragically—she didn't say how.

So many people had things to say and everyone listened to the speaker and looked at one another with such kindness, even though they didn't know them. There was great compassion in the room as people listened to the grief of another human being.

On my way home, I thought about all the different people that spoke, their losses and their sadness. I didn't think at all about myself, and there was such a feeling of largeness, because all these people had touched me. I connected with them all. The masters always talk about how the Lord needs space, and you have to make yourself wide and large, or the Lord can't really get in. I felt that was the case in the synagogue.

Then, I thought, "Well, how did the Lord get in there?" There was a lot of pain in that room, and through the heart, we connect. But, through a broken heart, we connect as well. And in that broken heart, we're all alike. It gives you the sense of humanity. Everyone in that room had had a broken heart, and there was a great feeling of togetherness and the Lord in that room. We shy away sometimes from pain—our own and others. But here there was no mistaking it.

My father didn't fast that year on Yom Kippur, and got mad at me for asking if he was. He said that at the age of eighty-seven he was too old. He told me, "Your mother's fasting and I told her not to, but she doesn't listen to me, so what can I do?" And then I really wished I had gone home to see my parents.

But, if I had, I wouldn't have been able to tell this story.

Once Upon a Time

हस्तस्य भूषणं दानं सत्यं कण्ठस्य भूषणम् ।
श्रोत्रस्य भूषणं शास्त्रं भूषणैः किं प्रयोजनम् ॥

hastasya bhūṣaṇaṃ dānaṃ satyaṃ kaṇṭhasya bhūṣaṇam
śrotrasya bhūṣaṇaṃ śāstraṃ bhūṣaṇaiḥ kiṃ prayojanam

The hand's ornament is charity. The neck's is truth. The ear's ornament is listening to knowledge. So what is the use of ornaments?

—FROM *THE SUBHASITANI*

Once upon a time, there was a man walking in the woods up on the mountains and he saw a group of students and their teacher sitting underneath a tree. There was such a sweet atmosphere around them that he wanted to get near them. He approached them, they welcomed him, and he sat down. The teacher continued teaching. The teacher was talking about kindness and the subtlety of existence. The man was excited to hear these words of the teacher. He felt that it was the most important thing that he had ever heard. He felt that the teacher's words were good words. He knew everything the teacher was saying, but somehow had forgotten it. By hearing the teacher speak about kindness, he could feel it within himself. He felt such relief. He asked himself, "How did I know to walk this way today, and come upon this beautiful teaching?"

This type of relief is called *samadhi.* It's a special state of mind where we remember what is most important. It's sometimes called an awakening, since it suggests that before we experienced *samadhi,* we were sleeping.

* * *

I was at a subway station, waiting for the train, and I saw a Japanese man playing an instrument with one string. He looked so gentle. The string had a beautiful echo and the man was singing, too. I gave him money. By doing this, I honor my teachers. I don't need to bring them fancy gifts. If I can give some money to the man in the subway playing songs, I honor my teachers just as well. Those are the teachings they gave me: to be responsive.

Ants Carrying Carrots

ॐ तच्छं योरावृणीमहे गातुं यज्ञाय गातुं यज्ञपतये दैवी स्वस्तिरास्तु नः
स्वस्तिर्मनुषेभ्यः ऊर्ध्वं जिगातु भेषजम् शं नौ अस्तु द्विपदे शं चतुष्पदे ॥
ॐ शन्तिः शन्तिः शन्तिः

oṃ tacchaṃ yorāvṛṇīmahe gātuṃ yajñāya gātuṃ yajñapataye
daivī svastirastu naḥ svastirmanuṣebhyaḥ ūrdhvaṃ jigātu
bheṣajam śaṃ nau astu dvipade
śaṃ castuṣpade oṃ śāntiḥ, śāntiḥ, śāntiḥ

I pray to the Lord that all of God's creatures who are relatives of mine, those with two legs and those with four legs, should be incredibly happy even after death.

—FROM *THE SHANTIH MANTRAS,*
THE GREAT PRAYERS FOR PEACE

People always ask my teacher, "What is yoga?" He says, "Yoga is union with God. That is all. That is all." Then he storms out of the room. The scriptures tell us that God is living in the hearts of all beings, that God is everywhere; that when we read a book, or go to a lecture, or attend a yoga class, or even when we get out of bed in the morning, there's something that we're looking for. The masters say that whatever we think it is, it's God. We might think it's our keys, but it's not.

I've gone to India for many summers to study yoga. In the beginning, one of the things that I found difficult was that there wasn't a separation between the outdoors and indoors. In America, we have windows and screens and houses made from solid material, so insects, worms, frogs, birds, pigeons, and squirrels, which live outside, never come inside. We have systems that keep animals outside, which we feel is their place. In India, they don't have that. What is outside can come inside and walk around, and then go back outside. It's not unusual to see a cow inside the post office. You think people would complain, but nobody does. I used to find this difficult.

Inevitably, you have all kinds of animals living in your house. You may have two hundred ants in your kitchen. I had this system, which I had learned from others, where you take all of your food, and put it in a metal tin, with a tight lid. Then you take that container, and put it in a bigger container full of water. The ants can't swim. So they make their way from the outside through the window along the kitchen counter, then up the outside of the bigger container and down the inside, and then they're stuck because there's a great big lake there, and they can't swim across. They circle around, and you feel sorry for them.

Even though I had this system, sometimes a grain of sugar would get left behind on the kitchen counter, and the ants would arrive. My desire was an ant-less kitchen. And so one day . . . I killed them. I killed all of them. And while I was killing them, I was aware of a conflict inside of me, but I worked hard not to be aware of it. I tried to be numb. There was something stirring in me, but I didn't pay attention to it. I went on with my day.

Then one day, I made a salad. I saw a piece of shredded carrot, about three inches long, moving along the kitchen floor, up the wall, and out the window. I looked closely, and saw about ten ants underneath carrying the carrot. We think of a shredded piece of carrot as a small thing, but if you're an ant, it's big and long and you need help from the other ants to carry it wherever you want to take it. There was this incredible teamwork going on and I didn't want to kill them. I just observed with a kind of gentleness.

From that day on, I stopped killing ants. If my guru was standing there, I would never have killed those ants; but since he wasn't there, I killed them, and that was a conflict in me. But from that day on, I stopped killing ants.

Yoga is union. There is no longer any conflict. You can wear a *mala* or set of beads, eat one meal a day, and have few things, but if you're killing ants, you'll be conflicted and life will be complicated. Tenderness keeps life simple. Lord Krishna teaches this when he says, "I am everywhere."

Do a Dirty Job

How do we learn humility? Only by putting ourselves in the field and doing honest hard work. Don't just sit and meditate or stand on your head for an hour at a time. Your ego will be boosted if you stand on your head that long. It is when you put your hand in the mud and do a dirty job that you will learn to be humble. Humility is the greatest virtue. It shows the purity of the mind.

—SWAMI SATCHIDANANDA

There is an ashram in upstate New York called Ananda Ashram, where I like to go. There is a swami there who is in her seventies named Ma Bhaskarananda, or Ma Bha for short. She was a disciple of Shri Brahmananda Saraswati for forty years and has lived at this ashram since she was a young woman. She wears orange robes, and has long gray hair that she wears in a thick braid. She has a child-like quality, a sparkle in her eye, and a space in between her two front teeth that you see when she smiles. I'm very fond of her and, whenever I see her, I bow down and she laughs that I bow. But I always do.

A couple of years ago I was up at the ashram leading a retreat with my husband. I drove in on a Friday and parked the car. On Monday, I was leaving by myself for New Hampshire, but was slow getting out of there, saying all my goodbyes and packing up, and by the time I was ready to go everyone else had left. When I went to my car, one of my tires was completely flat, and I thought, "What am I going to do?" I was totally flustered.

Then I looked up and saw Ma Bha with her ponytail and orange robes walking through the field. She must have sensed that I was flustered, so she came over and said, "What's wrong?"

I said, "I have a flat tire."

"Oh, is that all?"

"Yes." I replied.

"Well, do you have any tools?"

"I don't know."

"Well, do you have a spare tire?" she asked.

"I don't think so."

"Let's open up the trunk," Ma Bha said.

The trunk was full of stuff. She moved the stuff, and then lifted up the floor of the trunk. I didn't even know you could lift it up. Underneath was a tire and tools. "Oh, you have the tire," Ma Bha says. "You have the tools."

It had been raining all weekend and she—in her robes, in the mud, in her seventies, a Sanskrit scholar—changed my tire. I had always thought of her as being holy, pure, and virtuous, someone I'd like to be like. When I saw her on the ground, in the mud, changing my tire, she never looked more perfect to me. I was impressed beyond the beyond.

That is what Swami Satchidananda is saying: "Don't just stand on your head." It is good that we all have our practices. Human beings need practices—that is why they are there. But the practices should not be to serve the ego. The practices should lead us to serve each other. That's why participation is essential for *samadhi*.

What Can I Do?

यस्मान्नोद्विजते लोको लोकान्नोद्विजते च यः ।
हर्षामर्षभयोद्वेगैर्मुक्तो यः स च मे प्रियः ॥१५॥

yasmān nodvijate loko lokān nodvijate ca yaḥ
harṣāmarṣa-bhayodvegair mukto yaḥ sa ca me priyaḥ

The one who is not afraid of the world, and who the world is not afraid of, is dear to me.

—*THE BHAGAVAD GITA*, CHAPTER TWELVE, VERSE 15

We live in a beautiful world, where life is precious. We are blessed to be in this world. Still, there is so much violence. When you get deep into your yoga practice, your awareness and sense of affection increases, and because of that you ask yourself, "Is there something I can do to minimize the violence?" As your yoga practice deepens, this question persists. It's not like once in a blue moon, you wonder. It becomes a part of you. It's there, persisting. "What can I do? How can I bring harmony?"

I had an experience one summer in India. I was making many long-distance phone calls to America, because my father is in his mid-eighties, and I like to keep in touch with him. Also, my husband gets depressed when I'm gone all summer, so I like to call him regularly. There are many different places in India where you can go to make an overseas call, and one place belongs to my friend Shakunthala. For many years I've been going to her tiny shop to use the phone. When I go there, we chit chat and she makes tea. (There's another place that costs much less, it's half the price. But I don't think it's legal. It's not through the government. You actually go into somebody's home, where there is a computer hookup.)

This particular summer, I had an idea. Where I stay, everybody is Hindu, including my friends and teachers. But there's a Muslim section that's a little further removed from where I stay. I had a feeling that maybe I should go into the Muslim section and use the phone there. Since I didn't have any Muslim friends, maybe I could make some. It was a small thing, but it felt quite important.

So, I went off to the Muslim section, looking for a phone place, and found one. Inside was an older man who runs the shop with his family. He was wearing traditional Muslim clothing, and had beads and a little hat. I said, "I want to call America, can I go ahead?"

"Yes," he replied.

I thought I'd try and become friends with this man, whose name I learned was Atik.

On Father's Day, I called my dad, and when I got off the phone, I said to Atik, "We have this tradition in our country called Father's Day where we honor our fathers. I wanted to make sure to call my dad on this day."

"Oh, yes," Atik responded. "Father's Day is good. We have a custom like that, too, where we honor our fathers, we honor our parents, we honor the elderly people. This is good that you have that. We have that, too." We had this in common, Atik and I.

Another day, I told him I was calling my husband, Robert, because he gets depressed when I'm out of town.

Atik said, "Yes. I worked in Saudi Arabia for six years, and had to leave my wife, seeing her rarely." He said he was very depressed to be separated from her, so we also had that in common. He knew what it was like to be apart from your spouse, how you miss them. He understood completely.

We became very good friends, Atik and I. For ten weeks, I used his phone many times. His wife and daughters were usually in the back—they're modest under their veils—but they would peek out, and I would wave. They would smile at me, and I felt that I was their friend, too.

Sometimes I would be on the phone and he would bring me a tray of tea and cookies. I'd be talking to Robert and dipping my cookies in the tea. This friendship was peaceful and good.

When I was leaving India, I wanted to take some sweets to the family and say "goodbye." In India, people are very hospitable, and always bring gifts. It's a nice tip. Anytime you go anywhere, bring something: sweets, flowers. It's a beautiful way to live. I learned not to show up empty-handed, mostly.

So I brought sweets and said to Atik, "I'm an American and a Jew and you're a Muslim, and there's violence between these groups in the world; but that we have such a good rapport I feel is meaningful." I was choked up, and felt vulnerable, speaking to this Muslim man, who was old enough to be my father, and telling him these quirky insights that I was having. I was a little nervous confiding in him, telling him what's deep in my heart, how I felt that our relationship mattered on a global level. I didn't know how he would react.

He said to me, "Yes, I know exactly what you mean. I know exactly what you mean." He said he had many customers who are Hindu. Because the Hindus and Muslims also fight, he felt honored when the Hindus came into his shop. He liked that very much. He said even Pakistani people came to his shop. (The Indians and the Pakistanis are continuously fighting over the borderline. If you have a Pakistani stamp in your passport, and show up in India, the border guards can be rather unfriendly.)

Atik said, "Yes, I feel that we're keeping the peace, we're bringing harmony, I know exactly what you mean." He kept saying that he really understood what I meant. The two of us saw each other, the humanness and godliness of each other.

When I returned to New York City, I went to a little store on my street corner. The owners are from Yemen, and they sell cigarettes and coffee and newspapers. I go in there sometimes to get Alka-Seltzer. You can get one packet for fifty cents.

I like to go into the store. We live on the block together. Once I ran into the owner, way on the other side of the avenue, far away from the store. I wasn't sure he would know who I was out of context. But immediately he lit up, smiled, and said, "Hello." It was a small word, but special.

Where I live, New York City, people come from all over the world. This may be true wherever you live: Every neighborhood contains people with many different and wonderful backgrounds and experiences, if only we stopped to pay attention to them and said "Hello." On the microcosmic scale, if we could seize the opportunity to be at peace with each other, see each other, be friends with each other, and bring things to each other, we would see the effect worldwide.

Not Knowing When Death Occurs

प्रयाणकाले मनसाचलेन भक्त्या युक्तो योगबलेन चैव ।
भ्रुवोर्मध्ये प्राणमावेश्य सम्यक्स तं परं पुरुषमुपैति दिव्यम् ॥ १० ॥

prayāṇa-kāle manasācalena bhaktyā yukto yoga-balena caiva
bhruvor madhye prāṇam āveśya samyak sa taṃ
paraṃ puruṣam upaiti divyam

It's good to be thinking of God at the moment of death.

—*THE BHAGAVAD GITA*, CHAPTER EIGHT, VERSE 10

The Lord says that if you want to live a good and meaningful life, you have to consider death, because death is part of life. He says that you should have a good death, just like you should have a good life, and in order for that to happen, your mind should be at peace at the time of your death. He says that if you are not at peace, in your journey after death you will not find him easily. But on the other hand, if you have a good death, the next verse says, you will come to him easily, you will reach paradise. And in your next life, you could not ask for anything better. So according to the teachings of *The Bhagavad Gita*, our state of mind when we die determines what happens to us afterwards.

Whether or not you believe in reincarnation, or have thought about these things, or whether you believe in heaven and hell, or maybe you're not sure—or maybe you adopted your parent's beliefs—from what I've seen of death, everybody wants to go peacefully. I've seen many people who hadn't given much thought to being peaceful during their lives, but when death was looming, suddenly being peaceful was most important. Those of us with elderly parents want them to go peacefully. It would be terrible if my dad were upset about things at the time of his death. This is what Lord Krishna is saying.

Some time ago, I was angry with a friend of mine whom I love dearly. She had done many things to upset me. So I wrote her a letter that reflected my anger. I write well and can choose my words in a crafty manner. When I was done, I read it over to see what it was I had created. I thought it was quite good, and with that pumped-up feeling of satisfaction, I put that letter in an envelope, licked it shut, and took it to her assistant to deliver it.

Luckily, I did not die after that. I had an acupuncture appointment with an elderly, Japanese man, named Kenji Murata. He started out when he was twelve years old, cleaning the floor of his uncle's acupuncture clinic. It was there that he developed an interest in acupuncture. He noticed that people always left his uncle's office happy, and thought, "Wouldn't it be great to have a job where you could be of service like that?" He studied medicine and acupuncture diligently for many years so he could learn to heal people. Murata had a special way, a gentleness and humility, and there was a certain light around him.

He said to me, "I've been an acupuncturist for fifty years, and many people have come to me. All these people who come, they're so nice. I've met so many nice people." He started telling me about some of them, of the kind things they did, and how good-hearted they are. He said he couldn't believe how all these wonderful people had come into his life, and had touched him because of his work. I thoroughly enjoyed hearing this. I could feel his gratitude for having met all these nice people. It warmed my heart tremendously.

I went home and started thinking that, in my job as a yoga teacher, I'd also met many kind people. I felt blessed. I started picturing my students one by one. Then I remembered that letter, and thought about how it was so angry and wasn't even in my possession anymore. So, I called my friend's assistant, and she hadn't yet delivered the letter. I said, "Please, tear it up. Tear it up."

I started to think about the many positive ways that I could use words to deal with this situation. I'm a very creative and resourceful person. We all are. We are not always told that, but we are. We can solve our problems with a peaceful mind and a warm heart, instead of with negativity, and go beyond reactionary behavior, seeking alternative ways to approach our problems.

We don't know when we're going to die. I can hear my teacher's voice saying, "We never know, we never know." He would repeat it many times, giving examples of how we could be gossiping and then walk out the door, cross the street, get hit by a car, and die. We never know. Guruji would put the fear of death in us to help us get the point, because we think we'll be around forever, and we don't prepare, we don't think about it. I'm sure everybody knows someone who died suddenly. Lord Krishna is saying you want to die when your heart is warm, not cold. He is encouraging us to examine the contents of our minds and hearts every moment, so that we will always be ready to die.

A Mother's Love

मैत्रीकरुणामुदितोपेक्षणां सुखदुःख
पुण्यापुण्यविषयाणां भावनातश्चित्तप्रसादनम् ॥ ३३ ॥

maitrī karuṇā muditopekṣanāṃ sukha duḥkha
puṇyāpuṇyā viṣayāṇām bhāvanātaś citta prasādanaṃ

For those who are happy, you are happy too; you love them.

For those who are suffering, you want to take their pain away, you want to give them good things, you want to make them happy.

For those who are virtuous, you are joyful like a bright light.

For those who are wicked, you love them too, you don't want to hurt them, you just want to take their wickedness away. Through practices of loving-kindness our minds become crystal-clear, like pure water or blessed food.

—MASTER PATANJALI'S *YOGA SUTRAS*,
BOOK ONE, SUTRA 33

If we want to have a mind that is well—calm, not sick; clear and uncluttered rather than nervous—then there is a certain attitude toward others that we must follow. Master Patanjali says that if we see someone who is suffering, we should have compassion for that person, and not be hard-hearted or callous. You shouldn't pretend that you don't see them, or think, "Why don't they just get it together?"

In 2001, my mother wrote a memoir. It was about a period in her life when she was ten years old and living in Berlin. It was

1939, she was Jewish, and that September the Second World War broke out. My mother explains how one day the synagogues in the city were on fire, including the one where she went regularly for worship, and it was very frightening.

When she awoke the next morning, my mother discovered that her father had left for America and that her mother was preparing to leave for Czechoslovakia. Before leaving, my grandmother packed my mother a little suitcase and pushed her onto a train to Holland by herself.

So, my mother at the age of ten went with this little suitcase to Holland, where an English family picked her up and took her to England, where she stayed for six years. She was able to do this through a foster program where English families took refugee children from Nazi Germany and housed them.

In her memoir, my mother writes a little about the charmed life she left behind. She came from an extremely wealthy, high-society family. They lived in an old building with marble floors. The silverware they ate with was real silver; the tablecloths were made from fine linens; and the famous German painter Max Beckmann painted portraits of everyone in the family, which were framed in real gold. My mother said there was one nanny to braid the right side of her hair and another to braid the left. Her parents were very well-known. They had a box at the opera, and my grandmother was considered the best-dressed woman in all of Berlin. She never gained or lost more than two pounds, and always kept her figure.

My mother wrote that her family would have midday meals where everybody would gather: the uncles, aunts, nieces, nephews—sometimes there would be eighteen people sitting at the table. Even the servants would sit with the family. The meal would start with fruit soups and end with rhubarb pie. And in between were dishes such as white asparagus with hollandaise sauce. Such was the sophistication and harmony of the life my family had in Berlin that came to this very abrupt end.

My mother's memoir relates what it was like in England. The house she stayed in was in the countryside, which was very alien to her, since she'd grown up in Berlin. She tells of her fear of cows and pigs and other animals. The house, in a big field in the middle of nowhere, was exposed on all four sides, so the wind whipped around it. Her room was unfurnished, dark, cold, and damp. She would be sent by the family to walk six miles to get bread from the nearest farm, and the woman who sold the bread had Down's syndrome, and scared my mother.

Sometimes there wasn't money for food, and so my mother didn't know when the next meal was coming. She was entitled to one bath a week and the water was measured at three inches high. If you wanted to have hot water for your bath, you needed pennies to put into a little machine, and my mother had almost no pennies. She never saw many of her friends and family again and contracted meningitis and tuberculosis. She had a lot of hardships.

When I read my mother's book, I knew of the hardships she had experienced in her life, but not to the extent that I was finding out. I realized that my mother had held back in explaining what she had gone through as a child. I have had hardships, too, but none that compare to hers or others who come from places where there's been war. I myself have never had to flee from my home, seen my synagogue ablaze, wondered where my father was, or not known where my next meal would come from. I have not had meningitis.

Throughout my forty-some years of life, whenever I've had a hardship, I have frequently gone to my mother, and said something like, "Oh mother, please let me tell you my woes." And my mother has always said to me, "Oh, I don't want to see you suffer. What can I do for you? How can I heal you? What can I give to you? If I could take this away from you, I would. I would have it myself if I could save you from suffering." She has never said to me, "Look! I had to walk six miles. Maybe there would be bread there, maybe not. I needed pennies if I wanted hot water for my bath, and I had none. What are you complaining for? These things are trivial." She has never done that. She has always been so compassionate and loving.

I think my mother, because of everything she went through, is a wise person, and that when I've come to her with some kind of woe, she does not see just me—Ruth, her daughter with a problem—but is connected to the suffering of all beings, and I am just a part of the collective suffering that goes on in the universe. There is always suffering going on in each one of us and in the world.

So when I complain to her, she immediately feels the greater suffering of humanity, and because of that she has a universal compassion. It is always healing to go to her. We can do this for ourselves. When we are suffering, for whatever reason, we can bring it out of the egotistical arena and feel that the suffering we're having, others are having, too. When we can rise above the prison of our ego, and feel the suffering of mankind, then instead of closing down, we open up. That opening leaves its mark on you, and makes you a better human being.

* * *

My acupuncturist, Kenji Murata, was a master, a healer, and a great human being. Acupuncture is a bit like a yoga class, in that the treatment is painful, but I always leave feeling great. When I went to see him, I tried not to complain and let him do his work, but sometimes the pain was too great to keep quiet. So I said to him, "It hurts. I'm in pain."

Murata would see two people at once. A Japanese screen divided the room where he practiced. He said, "Yes, the man next to you, he is in pain, also. I have so many patients, they are all in pain."

I was lying there thinking that I was the only one in pain. And when he said, "But the man on the other side of the screen is in pain, too," I thought about that man, and all the people who go to a doctor of some sorts because they're in pain and need to be touched. Immediately, I felt relief from thinking only of myself.

Ram's Greatest Quality

श्री राम् जै राम् जै जै राम्

Śrī Rām, Jai Rām, Jai Jai Rām

Hail, hallelujah, and victory to the Lord Ram.

—A CHANT TO LORD RAM

Once upon a time, there was a god named Ram. Ram was said to be a very great god, with many good qualities. Some people said Ram had ninety-nine good qualities. Other people said, "No, Ram has 108 good qualities." Still other people claimed that he had 84,000, and yet others said his good qualities were immeasurable and innumerable. In any case, we can say that Ram had a lot of good qualities!

Sometimes the *pandits*, yogis, pilgrims, and scholars would get together and discuss what the greatest of all the good qualities of Ram was, and concluded that the best quality was that Ram always introduced himself to anyone. If he saw the king, he would say to himself, "Oh! I'm going to say 'hello' to the king." If he saw a beggar, he would think, "Oh! I'm going to say 'hello' to the beggar." If he saw somebody with his nose up in the air that wasn't interested in saying 'hello,' Ram would conclude, "He may be a difficult one, but I want to say 'hello'." He wouldn't wait for the other to say "hello" first. He did not have that kind of smallness or pride. He lived his life this way. He made friends with everyone, from all different walks of life, and he was completely at home in the world. This was said to be his greatest quality.

One month, I led a retreat in the countryside. Many students from New York City came. Most of them had been on retreats before, and they were all friends with each other, so they didn't need to introduce themselves, and it was easy for them to be together. However, there was one lady who, though she comes to my class regularly, keeps to herself. So, as the years have passed, she hasn't gotten to know people.

Early on in the retreat, I welcomed her and asked her how the retreat was going. She said, "Well, I feel kind of weird, because I don't know any of these people. They all know each other, and I feel separate from the group. I was looking forward to coming, but now I feel awkward. Maybe I should go back to New York City."

I said, "Well, dear student, do you know the story of Ram?" She didn't, and so I told it to her.

The next day at lunch, I saw her go up to a table of people and introduce herself. She said, "May I sit with you?" Everybody smiled and moved over. "I'm happy to meet you," she said. For the next two days, every time I saw her, instead of being alone she was with others. It is so important to be engaged with others. It's called intimacy. If you don't know others, you won't know yourself.

By the end of the retreat, this woman was touching the others with handshakes or hugs. There was a heaviness about her that had been lifted. It's a beautiful way to live your life, being always ready to say "hi." If you go about your days with this sentiment toward your fellow beings, after a time you'll have the sense that something deep inside of you is changing. The sense of things being burdensome lifts . . . and you're ready to mingle with the world.

The Chewed-Up Cat

सर्वे भवन्तु सुखिनः सर्वे सन्तु निरामयाः
सर्वे भद्राणि पश्यन्तु मा कश्चित् दुःखभाग्भवेत्

sarve bhavantu sukhinaḥ sarve santu nirāmayāḥ
sarve bhadrāṇi paśyantu mā kaścit duḥkha bhāgbhavet

May all be happy. May all be free from sickness.
May all see what is good and beautiful. May no one be unhappy.

—A TRADITIONAL PRAYER BEFORE CLASS

I've developed this habit of going into a pet store. They have a program where you can adopt a cat or kitten right in the store. Twenty to thirty cats are in cages and the hope is that someone will adopt them. The first few times I went, I noticed the kittens. They were around eight weeks old, so everything was new to them. They were cute, sweet, and cuddly, and I thought maybe I'd take one home, and put him or her on my lap. I went home and told my husband Robert about the kittens, and that maybe I'd bring one home.

"Fine," he said.

I started going every day, and it became sort of an obsession. After about ten days, I noticed that the kittens would come and go, and there was a turnover. Smoochy was there on Sunday, and gone on Monday. Somebody had taken her. Kittens go quickly. I noticed that the older cats had been in the store for many days, while the kittens, batches of them, had come and gone. I could see that these slightly older cats were sad. Maybe the average person thinks they're slightly less cute and cuddly. It was depressing. They had their food and litter boxes and beds all within a tiny cage in the store, far away from the windows.

I thought it would be better to take one of these older cats. It would be more compassionate. I went home and asked Robert, "Can we take one that's six months old? They're more sad and they get stuck in the store."

"Fine," he said.

I went back the next day. There was an eight-year-old cat who had been mistreated, abandoned, and couldn't stop chewing things. He had chewed his bed, the litter box, and half his hair off, and he was chewing on the bars of the cage. The cat looked like this overactive, tired-out, chewed-up little creature. When I asked the lady about him she said that he didn't have a name and that no one would adopt him because he chewed everything up.

I thought, this cat is suffering more than any of the other cats, and it was heartbreaking. I went home and said to Robert, "There's this chewed-up, nameless cat who's really suffering that I'd like to adopt. It would be a rescue."

"Fine," he said.

So for nearly a month, I came home every other day with new news about which cat we were going to adopt. I was thinking that this reflects the process of *sadhana,* or spiritual practice. You start out concerned about the kittens, because they're cute and cuddly, and then your concern expands, and you consider that you could love the older cat as well. Then you see a cat that will be a challenge and chew everything up, and you think you could also love that cat.

In a similar way, you reach a point where you decide to be a vegetarian. If your cares are limited, then there's a lot that gets left uncared for. Caring for others, all others, is the foundation of a yoga practice. In yoga it's called *ahimsa,* or nonviolence, or *karuna,* compassion.

The Blessing of the Elder

उन्मन्यवाप्तये शीघ्रं भ्रूध्यानं मम संमतम् ।
राजयोगपदं प्राप्तुं सुखोपायोऽल्पचेतसाम् ।
सद्यः प्रत्ययसंधायी जायते नादजो लयः ॥ ८० ॥

unmanyavāptaye śīghraṃ bhrūdhyānaṃ mama sammatam
rājayogapadaṃ prāptuṃ sukhopāyo'lpacetasām
sadyaḥ pratyayasaṃdhāyī jāyate nādajo layaḥ

Contemplation on the eyebrow center leads to
universal vision that is truth bearing.

—*THE HATHA YOGA PRADIPIKA*, CHAPTER FOUR, VERSE 80

The *ajna chakra* is the fifth chakra from the bottom of the spine. Its location is the point between the two eyebrows, often called the third eye. Sometimes you see pictures of a yogi in meditation, or ancient paintings of deities, and there's a dot between the eyebrows. That's the *ajna chakra*. In yoga, the goal is to open that third eye. If that eye is open, we see things in a holy and tender way.

Ajna itself means wisdom, insight, or honey-like knowledge. If you have enough honey-like knowledge, you will never die. It's an elixir that is better than water.

My dear friend Shakunthala, who lives in India, had polio and was abandoned as a baby. She lived in various orphanages, or with foster parents, or on the street. She had a lot of hardship growing up.

When Shakunthala was a young adult, and still in the orphanage, one man sponsored her education, and she learned about computers. When she was finished with her schooling, she got a job and made money. The first thing she did with the money was to pay back the man who had sponsored her. He told her it was not necessary, but she wanted to pay him back, so he could sponsor someone else.

Some years passed, and she opened up a little shop with a computer, and offered help on the Internet. She also sold chocolate and cookies. When Shakunthala's mother became ill, all of the other siblings (who her mother had kept) were very busy and couldn't take care of their mother. So Shakunthala, in addition to her chores, started taking the bus every day, to go cook, clean, and look after her mother.

I said, "Shakunthala, you're taking care of a woman who abandoned you?"

She said, "Yes, she is my mother."

Shakunthala married a man, Girish, who is also handicapped, and she became pregnant. One day, after feeding the children at the orphanage, we were walking home together. It is very difficult for Skakunthala to walk—she has to drag her leg—but it's good for her to get exercise. This was especially so since she was pregnant. It was monsoon season and thundering. It was dramatic because we had just left the orphanage, and we were feeling emotional.

Shakunthala turned and said to me, "What will happen if I die in childbirth? My husband is also handicapped. Who will take care of my child?"

I said, "Shakunthala, you mustn't speak like that, you're young, you have a good doctor."

"No," she insisted. "I'm not young. You're young." Even though I'm fifteen years older than Shakunthala, my life has had less hardship than hers, and I do look younger.

She said, "You come here, and you study with your teacher. He is a holy man."

I'm always talking to her about my teacher, how holy, pure, and perfect he is. She said, "If I could meet him, have the blessing of the holy pure man just once, the blessing of the elder, then I will not die in childbirth. Can you arrange that I meet your teacher?"

Then thunder and lightning crashed. This was the only thing she had ever asked me for in all the years of our friendship and I could feel the depth of her request. I wanted to do what she was asking.

In India, there are codes and traditions that are set down and very old, and have to do with the caste system. I knew that Shakunthala was not the same caste as my guru. She's a local person and I rarely see local people in my guru's house. The only people I ever see there are his students or his relations. I didn't want to do anything incorrect. My teacher has already given me the teachings of yoga, so to ask for extra is something I have never done. I was unsure what to do. But in the end I honored my friend's request.

Early the next day, I went into my teacher's office. "Guruji," I said. "My friend is a good woman, she's feeding the children in the orphanage, and has one bad leg. She's going to have a baby and wants to have your blessing. Can she come to see you?"

Guruji said, "HUH?!" He made me repeat the whole thing. Then he said, "What is her name?"

"Shakunthala."

"Oh. She is living where?"

"8th Cross, Guruji."

"Oh, 8th Cross. One flour mill is there."

"Yes, Guruji. Her husband is related to that flour mill man."

"Oh, flour mill man family. Yes. When do you want to come?"

I said, "Can we come tomorrow?"

"Yes, tomorrow you come. You bring that lady, no problem."

I went running to Shakunthala and said, "Tomorrow we can go."

Shakunthala's poor, but she has one nice dress and she wanted to buy flowers.

I said, "I'll buy the flowers."

"Oh no," she responded. "I'm purchasing the flowers." Of course, she bought many flowers.

We took the flowers to Guruji's office. Shakunthala and Guruji began speaking in Kannada, which is one of the languages of southern India, so I didn't even know what they were talking about. They spoke for a long time and I was full of joy.

Then Guruji turned and said to me, "Your friend is very good, she is helping others. Not for name, not for name. So many people helping others only for name's sake. She is quietly helping others. This is good woman." This is true. She is in her little corner helping others quietly, and that's who she is. He immediately picked up on it.

Then I said to my friend, "We should go." We had been in there for about twenty minutes. Shakunthala said, "Well, I want to get the blessing." So Shakunthala, with her bad leg, her whole body pushed askew because of it, and the difficulty she has in getting up and down, got down on the floor in full prostration, and bowed to my guru. Guruji was smiling and tapping her on the head.

When we left, Shakunthala said, "I will not die in childbirth and my child will be healthy. I have received the blessing of the elder, the holy man." Guruji had told her that she could come anytime, and I said, "Shakunthala, you can go anytime."

Shakunthala replied, "I've already received it. I don't need ever to go again. I've received the blessing."

I thought to myself, "I've received the blessing so many times." Because when you get to Guruji's center you receive a blessing; and after class you get another blessing; and then if you linger around, which I always do, you get still another blessing. If you're there for a few months, that adds up to a lot of blessings. It was through Shakunthala's eyes that I was able to see the blessing in a different light. Even though I would never take the blessing for granted, when I saw what it meant to her, it made me see my blessing with more gratitude and humility.

* * *

My friend Jane, who does a lot of volunteer work in Darfur, sees what the world is like for many people who are refugees and victims of violence. When she returns home to New York, and crawls into her clean, safe, and large bed, she sees it differently, because of what she has experienced in Darfur. Sometimes vision is like that. We have to see it through the eyes of someone else, and not feel limited to our own two eyes . . . when there is a third eye.

Man Cannot Live on Bread Alone

मत्तः परतरं नान्यत्किञ्चिदस्ति धनञ्जय ।
मयि सर्वमिदं प्रोतं सूत्रे मणिगणा इव ॥ ७ ॥

mattaḥ parataraṃ nānyat kiñcid asti dhanañjaya
mayi sarvam idaṃ protaṃ sūtre maṇi-gaṇā iva

All beings in the world are strung on the Lord as pearls on a thread.
Once you are able to see God in the beautiful and the sacred,
then you start to see God everywhere. Like beads on a necklace,
or rays of the sun, we are all children of God.

—*THE BHAGAVAD GITA*, CHAPTER SEVEN, VERSE 7

Once when I was in San Francisco, I visited some friends who have a yoga center in the city. They were giving a class on vegan cooking and invited me to come. I'm always looking for new recipes, especially for my husband, so I took the class. The money raised from the class fee would be used to make a meal on Thanksgiving for a local soup kitchen. They suggested a donation price for the class. Even though I don't live in San Francisco, and wouldn't be there on Thanksgiving, and wouldn't need to go to a soup kitchen for my meal, I wanted to give a donation.

After the class, I went to a service for a friend of mine who had passed away from cancer. She was a great dancer, a master of what is called "Odissi" dance, which comes from the Orissa region of India, and has a lot of intricate footwork. It looks easy, but in fact it's very difficult. My friend spent twenty-three years in India learning this technique. At the service, they were collecting money for a trust in her name, so those wanting to go abroad and study this type of dance could go. I wanted to give a donation.

After visiting San Francisco, I went to San Diego, where some friends of mine have a yoga center. After class, I was in the dressing room and saw a flyer posted on the wall describing an upcoming workshop. The purpose of the workshop was to raise money for a student in their community with cancer who had no medical insurance. Even though I couldn't take the workshop, I went to the lady at the front desk and registered for it.

She said, "But you're not going to be here."

"Well, that's OK. I'd like to make a donation."

"Yes, but you won't be here," she repeated.

"Yes, but I'd like to," I said.

On my way back to New York, there was a kid standing in front of me at the airport, dressed like a soldier. I couldn't believe he was a soldier because he looked like a child. He had braces and pimples, and was chubby like I was at that age. When we had to show our IDs, I saw he had a special ID for the military. The security guard that he handed his ID to said, "Thank you for serving. Take care over there."

"Thank you," he said.

Immediately I thought, "Gosh, I wish him well. He's just a kid. I hope everything goes OK for him." Then I thought, "Whoever he thinks his enemy is, I wish them well, too."

On the plane, I recalled a friend of mine, who has a sick friend. I had been calling her during the week to ask how her friend was and could tell from the sound of her voice that her friend wasn't doing well. I've never met her friend, but I knew her name, and it kept coming up in my mind. I kept thinking of this woman and her name.

In these ways, you connect yourself to everybody. "Yoga" means "to join." It doesn't happen overnight, that feeling of being connected to all people, but it starts to unfold through the practices of yoga. In *The Bhagavad Gita,* the Lord says to his student, "I am everywhere. I am in all people. I am in all beings. I am everything. I am in front of you, behind you, to the right of you, to the left of you. I am everybody's grandfather."

When we feel connected to everyone, really we're connected to the Lord. Otherwise, it's like, "I don't know the people at the soup kitchen, I don't care about the arts, I don't have cancer, and I don't believe in this war." When we're self-absorbed and cut off from others, really we're cut off from God. If we're cut off from God, it leads to profound malnourishment and we'll always be hungry. Bad habits arise out of hunger. Disorders, compulsive behaviors, overindulgence, and greed all come from excessive hunger that can never be satisfied when we're cut off from God and his creatures.

In the Bible, it says, "Man cannot live on bread alone." This is a famous line. Often we take bread for granted, see it only as bread, and even let it go stale. But the bread is the wheat, the earth, the water, the air, the sun, the farmer, the baker, the merchant . . . all of that is the bread. All of that is the Lord. If you eat the bread and it's not connected to all of that, it is just bread: you cannot live on that bread alone. But if you see the bread as the earth, the water, the air . . . then the bread is sacred, and one piece is enough.

Carry It Through

नियतं कुरु कर्म त्वं कर्म ज्यायो ह्यकर्मणः ।
शरीरयात्रापि च ते न प्रसिद्ध्येदकर्मणः ॥ ८ ॥

niyataṃ kuru karma tvaṃ karma jyāyo hyakarmaṇaḥ
śarīra yātrāpi ca te na prasiddhyed akarmaṇaḥ

Anyone in the world needs to act. Even just to take care of one's body, one needs to act.

—*THE BHAGAVAD GITA*, CHAPTER THREE, VERSE 8

Once, I was in California visiting my parents. When I got to their house, I noticed that my father, who was 587 years old, was very much in need of a haircut. His hair was matted and it didn't seem like you could get a comb through it. His scalp was very dry and it was unpleasant to look at. I said, "Dad, I could take you for a haircut."

I thought he would put up a fight because he never leaves the house, but he seemed happy with the idea, and said, "Yes. There is a barber I know."

"I noticed there was an Aveda nearby," I added, "which is a salon that uses products made with plants and not chemicals. Your scalp looks like it could use some plant-based products and they have a good reputation." Again, I thought my father would put up a fight and say that a barber was good enough for him. But he thought those plant-based products sounded good.

I put him in the car, and drove slowly. We found a parking spot (Thank you, Lord!) right in front of the salon, and I carefully walked him in, and said to the lady at the front desk, "I would like my dad to have a haircut."

"It'll be ten minutes," she said. I was worried that my father would say he couldn't wait. But he was very agreeable, and said, "Fine."

We waited and in five minutes she took him and washed his hair. I said, "Be gentle with him," and she was. Afterwards, she asked my father what kind of shampoo he uses. He said he uses baby shampoo from CVS, which is a low-end drugstore.

She said, "Your shampoo could be the cause of the rashes on your scalp, which could become infected. You should use a shampoo and conditioner of a better quality."

The woman was very friendly, and suggested that we purchase a shampoo and a conditioner at the store. My father said he couldn't stand long enough in the shower to shampoo and condition on account of his age.

"Oh, it's no problem," said the woman. "Dump half of the shampoo out, fill it up with conditioner, mix it up, and do the same with the other bottle and then it will be all in one."

"I'll do that when we get home," I assured my father.

"OK," he responded.

My dad then went to the bathroom, which was good because then I could pay while he was gone. Even though the haircut and shampoo only cost $46, which I thought was reasonable, I knew my father would think anything above $12 was highway robbery. Also, I gave the hairdresser a good tip, because my father wouldn't have—not because he's stingy, but because he lives in a different era. When he came out of the bathroom, I thought he might ask about the fee but when I said, "We're ready to go," he said "OK."

My father used the shampoo a couple of times while I was there, and by the time I left, his hair and scalp looked much better. As an old man, his dignity is connected to the way he looks, and I think he was happy about the haircut. He doesn't get happy often, so it was nice to see. And I was glad, because whenever I visit my parents, I always want to do something, to be of help in some way. This was something.

Everybody needs help. I need help, you need help, people in your families need help, and the person who lives next door needs help. Where you work—your co-workers, your boss, people who work under you, above you, with you—they need help. The people you don't know, the people you will meet tomorrow, they will need help. Everybody needs help, and we're all here to help each other.

If you have an idea of how to help someone, but then you think, "Well, I'm busy," or "They're not worth it," or "They did a bad thing to me a while back," or "I'm just lazy," and you don't carry it through, that's when you stop growing spiritually. Where you stop helping others and where you stop growing is the same. If you have an idea of how to help someone, even if it's a small thing . . . carry it through.

An Arrogant Student

तद्विद्धि प्रणिपातेन परिप्रश्नेन सेवया ।
उपदेक्ष्यन्ति ते ज्ञानं ज्ञानिनस्तत्त्वदर्शिनः ॥३४ ॥

tad viddhi praṇipātena paripraśnena sevayā
upadekṣyanti te jñānaṃ jñāninas tattva-darśinaḥ

Go to the teacher, and sit at their feet. When you want to learn something, go to the wise one and bow down.

—*THE BHAGAVAD GITA*, CHAPTER FOUR, VERSE 34

When I am in India I take yoga classes. The room where classes are held holds fifty students. But at any given time, there are more than fifty students at the school, so students must practice in batches. Each person goes at his own pace and, when he's finished, another student takes his place. It's been like that for some time, except in the olden days when there were few people at the school.

When you first arrive, you pay and register and the teacher tells you what time to come. Sharath told me, "Come at 6:30."

I always set my clock fast when I'm in India by twenty-five minutes. I live two houses away from the school, so it takes less than a minute to get there. So between setting my clock fast and being so close, I was there at five after six, but I wasn't concerned.

I went in, and in the foyer were ten people waiting their turn. You can see into the classroom from the foyer through wide-open doors. I took my seat among the people and in less than a minute a spot inside the classroom opened up. I happened to see it. Sharath yelled out, "One more, come!" Nobody jumped up. They were laid back, and so I went in. I walked halfway through the room and I heard Sharath on the other side of the room yelling, "Ruth, no, no, no. You go back. Others are before you."

So I went back. I took my seat in the foyer among the others. I sat there and waited for everyone who had come before me to go, and only then did I take my spot. But as I was sitting there, I recollected being shouted at really loudly, "Ruth! You go back!" I took that in, and thought to myself how happy I was to be scolded. In his own way, Sharath was telling me, "Ruth, that part of you that thinks you can jump ahead of others or come whenever you want, I'm not impressed by that. It doesn't mean anything to me. That's not the subject we're studying. Take that wardrobe off. After you take that wardrobe off, *that's* what we're studying."

There is a way to be between student and teacher, and between student and student. If the teacher says come at 6:30, then come at 6:30. If the other students are ahead of you, don't put yourself ahead of them. There's a way to be all the time in the world with others, a mutually beneficial way to behave. We will not find the way, and will never know how to be, when the ego's first. That's why it helps to have a guru.

The Tong Len

आत्मौपम्येन सर्वत्र समं पश्यति योऽर्जुन ।
सुखं वा यदि वा दुःखं स योगी परमो मतः ॥ ३२ ॥

ātmaupamyena sarvatra samaṃ paśyati yo 'rjuna
sukhaṃ vā yadi vā duḥkhaṃ sa yogī paramo mataḥ

One who knows the sorrows and the happiness of others as his own is a perfect yogi. In other words, a devotee of the Lord always tends to the joys and sorrows of others, and in this way is a friend to everyone.

—*THE BHAGAVAD GITA*, CHAPTER SIX, VERSE 32

As you go deep into yoga practice and try to be a good practitioner, you tap into a wisdom that you're able to use. You find yourself often thinking about what good you could offer to the community. I'm amazed to see that in myself. Years ago, if I was sitting in a yoga class, and the teacher started talking about what we could do for others, I'd be uninterested. But, through these practices, you change, and see that you've been given some gifts, and whether they're large or small, they can be used to help others. This is how you know your practice is working.

I was at a Buddhist retreat at Diamond Mountain University in the middle of the Arizona desert, in a tent. We did a Buddhist meditation called Tong Len, which I had never done before. The man leading the meditation gave us instructions on what to do and how to do it. The first thing we were supposed to do was pick someone who was suffering. I knew so many people who were suffering, but one person stood out. Then the meditation leader said, "It helps to be very specific, and go through it in your mind."

The person I chose was one of the 300 people in the tent. She was swollen, and had little hands and feet, dark green rings under her eyes, and she was walking with a walker. I had noticed her during our short breaks. People would run out of the tent to go to the bathroom, get some water, and then run back in. It was difficult for her to make her way out of and back to the tent. Microphones were being used, and there were wires running along the ground that she could easily trip over. I could see that she was suffering. So I chose her.

Then the leader said we could relieve this person of their suffering by taking what they have for ourselves. It's a meditation, and he was asking us to repeat after him, "Give their suffering to me." I knew that the meditation wouldn't end there. But, when we got to that part, "Give it to me," I thought, "Gosh, I don't want what she has, the swelling, the rings under her eyes, the walker. . . ." The leader was saying, "Relieve that person from their suffering. Take it, swallow it, and see it going into your system." I couldn't do it. So I sat there and thought, "Well, this is as far as I go."

Some days passed, and the retreat ended. During the retreat, I had sung at the beginning of each session. Everybody thanked me for the singing, and said it was nice. On the last day, the woman I had chosen for the Tong Len meditation, came up close to me. I think she even took my hand. I felt very close to her, and she had sought me out. She said, "I want to thank you for the singing, and I want you to know how healing it was for me."

Everybody had thanked me for the singing, but nobody had used the word *healing*. And when she used that word *healing*, there was a sense of well being in the way that she said it, and she looked better. It made a big impression on me, and I realized that the Tong Len had worked, even though I couldn't complete it.

There was another retreat six months later. During those six months, I kept wondering how that woman was doing. The Tong Len had really carved a space in my heart for her, and when I went to the next retreat, she was the first person I wanted to see. However, she wasn't there, and nobody could tell me what had happened to her.

I want to encourage something as basic as noticing and caring when someone is suffering, and keeping them in mind.

Holy Objects

The student asked the question, "If one has a holy object from a saintly person, will that object keep the holy vibration forever?"

Shri Gurudev: "It depends upon how you keep it. If you keep it in the proper way, in the proper place, without polluting it, it will express holiness forever. But if you just leave it casually somewhere and don't treat it properly, slowly, it will lose its energy. As long as holy objects are kept with reverence and respect, as long as they are kept that way, they will emit holy vibration."

—A READING FROM SWAMI SATCHIDANANDA,
FROM *THE GOLDEN PRESENT*

I have this great music teacher in India, Dr. Gurudat, who has taught me many prayers. He knows thousands of them. Every day I ask, "Can I have a new prayer?"

"Oh yes!" he says. "Thousands are there. Which one do you want?" The number of prayers is vast.

Dr. Gurudat teaches music to children in his home and many of those children come from families who don't have extra money for music lessons. The parents negotiate the fee and because Dr. Gurudat wants the child to have music in their lives, he charges very little. He gives lessons to many children. He lives simply, and has very few material objects in his home. It's quite refreshing to see. If you want to sit down, he pulls out a straw mat. He has one pot for cooking rice and two shirts that hang on hooks. His home is full of children, and music, and prayers. It never feels poor. It feels rich. I love going over there.

One year, on the day of my last class, Dr. Gurudat said to me, "Ruth, today I want to present one gift to you." He was gleaming.

I said, "Oh, Guruji, you shouldn't be making presentations to me. I'm your student, I should be making presentations to you."

"Oh no!" he said. "Nothing doing. You are all the time bringing me gifts. Today, I will make my presentation to you. Sit."

Dr. Gurudat called for his wife, Chandrika, who is always in the kitchen. She came out of the kitchen, a little sweaty, and they began speaking to each other in the Kannada language. Then she opened up a drawer and brought out a box. She opened it, took out a bag, opened this, and removed a shawl. Dr. Gurudat looked happy and Chandrika came up to me, bowed, and presented me with this shawl.

In India, there are many different kinds of shawls and most Westerners and tourists buy fancy ones. When you go into a store, immediately the salesman shows you the ones made of cashmere or silk. Indians don't buy these shawls. The shawl that my teacher and his wife presented to me was a worker's shawl. I felt honored that they thought I was worthy of one of these. For me, that shawl was a holy object because it came from a family who took great satisfaction in the act of giving. To give me something satisfied them in a way that I think most of us never truly experience. I was overcome.

When I came back to New York, my husband, Robert, went rifling through my suitcase to see what treasures I had brought back from India. Without too much time, he got to that shawl. He put it on, and said, "Of all the things that you brought back from India, I want this."

I was so happy and said, "Yes! You look dashing in it. You shall have it. Take that shawl. It is holy."

We all have objects that come to us from time to time in some special way. The story behind the object is what gives the object its spiritual quality. When we have objects like that, it is good to savor the experience, the essence of the object. It's a refined emotion, to savor something. We might even cry. When I see Robert in the shawl, I could cry.

I've been a reader of the *New York Times* for many years. When I used to see full-page ads for Macy's "One Day Sale," they would grab my attention. Now, they don't. As you go deeper into your *sadhana,* you need fewer material objects. Shopping is not what you want to be doing with your holy life. That's a sign that your *sadhana* is working.

Reverence for the Totality of Creation

सर्वभूतस्थमात्मानं सर्वभूतानि चात्मनि ।
ईक्षते योगयुक्तात्मा सर्वत्र समदर्शनः ॥२९॥

sarva-bhūta-stham ātmānaṃ sarva-bhūtāni ca ātmani
īkṣate yoga-yuktātmā sarvatra sama-darśanaḥ

The yogi sees the Lord in all. We can bow to the Lord everywhere.

—*THE BHAGAVAD GITA*, CHAPTER SIX, VERSE 29

Once, my Sanskrit teachers from India visited New York City to teach, which was wonderful. I love and worship them and bow down to them often. I have pictures of them in my house and if people bring me flowers I put them by their pictures.

In this verse and in the yoga teachings, it's emphasized that when you worship or feel reverence for someone, you should not attach yourself to the personality or the body of the person you have reverence for. The body is changing and passing and material. Yoga is a spiritual practice. We are encouraged to look deeper than the body when worshipping the Lord. In this verse it's called the *atman,* the soul. That is what we should be worshipping. When we say "*Namaste,*" it is the soul that we bow down to.

Sama darshanah is to practice seeing the same soul in all beings. *Brahman,* the word for "God" in Sanskrit, means "always expanding." It's a very beautiful notion of God. If we have this reverence for the soul in our teachers, that should be always expanding, so that that reverence doesn't just stay for our teachers but goes to the totality of creation. That is what the yogi aims for, a vision of the Lord that is always expanding.

That type of vision comes as a result of yoga. You see sacredness in all of life. Then choices like vegetarianism come naturally, easily. You want to cause the least harm possible. You don't want to live a life where your happiness is at the expense of others. Of course, to some degree it always will be, but you want to minimize, minimize, minimize. It's a refinement, to go from gross to subtle, so that your footprint is less. Because of that, for the yogi to be a vegetarian, to not eat animals, takes no discipline at all. It takes discipline to wake up early, or not to eat too much sugar, or to study Sanskrit grammar. But to be a vegetarian, it's out of gentleness and out of love. Anything that comes from love is certainly palatable.

A Tinge of Sadness

तीव्रसंवेगानामासन्नः ॥ २१ ॥

tīvra saṃvegānām āsannaḥ

If our practice is intense and has speed, not mild and slow, then enlightenment will be nearby.

—MASTER PATANJALI'S *YOGA SUTRAS*, BOOK ONE, SUTRA 21

I think if you have the feeling that others will be affected positively by your practice, and not only you, it helps you to work seriously.

When I returned from India one time, I didn't feel well. I was anxious, and the anxiety was increasing. People picked up on it, and were tender with me. A friend of mine gave me a phone number of the acupuncturist, Kenji Murata. I called Murata up and left a message saying, "Dear doctor, I'm not feeling well. I hope I can come see you tomorrow. Please call me back."

He called me back and said, "Tomorrow is fine. What time can you come?"

"How would six o'clock be?" I replied.

"Fine, no problem. See you then."

Immediately, from the sound of his voice, and the fact that he called me back so promptly, I felt better.

The next day, I went to the acupuncturist's, and on my way I started to get a little nervous, because acupuncture can be intense. As I was climbing the stairs, I thought that perhaps I shouldn't be going. However, I went in and this man was so kind, he reminded me of my father. He had a quality of goodness that you cannot fake. I felt that I was at the right place. He gave me a treatment, I liked it, and I went back to see him once a week for five weeks in a row.

During the treatments, we didn't talk much. I didn't mind. I like quiet. Although we hardly spoke to each other, I felt a lot of love for him, and I could feel that he felt love for me, too.

Then one day I went to see him, and he was quite talkative. He said, "I'm helping so many people." Then he started telling me all the people that he had helped. "One lady wanted a baby. Five years of trying went by and still no baby. She was forty-three. I worked with her for five months and then, a baby. One man who works on a computer many hours a week had carpal tunnel. His fingers were stuck into his palms. He could not open up his hands. He couldn't even button his shirt. The doctor said he needed to have surgery, so he thought to try acupuncture instead. After five treatments, his hands opened, no need for surgery. I fixed it."

I could tell Murata was very happy to have saved this man from the pain of having surgery when it really wasn't needed.

"Another man had chronic fatigue syndrome," Murata continued. "He was sleeping all the time. His energy was blocked. After five treatments, his energy was circulating. I fixed it."

Murata told me of all the different people and their ailments, and what he had done for them. He did it with total humility, and without ego. It was simply that he'd had his hand in something good—that his work was meaningful. He put it very simply, but there was joy in his voice.

Then Murata added: "One patient had cancer. The cancer had spread, and it was too late. I couldn't fix it." He said it with such sadness, I was very moved. I think that he wouldn't have been as good a doctor if he had not really felt sad that he couldn't solve the person's condition. If he hadn't been such a good doctor, I don't think he would have called me back so quickly. I think he heard my pain, and it made him sad and he called me back immediately, so he could fix it.

There is a sensitivity that we have as human beings to feel each other's sadness. It keeps us connected, keeps us human. Often, we put so much emphasis on being happy, and pretend that we're not sad when we can't help somebody who has cancer. But our potential as human beings is to have a happiness that is so real that it has room in it for sadness. And that's why all the saints have a tinge of sadness in their faces. I've been lucky enough to see a few saints, and it's true. They have that sadness and sense of urgency, because people in the world are suffering, and it's out of that sadness and urgency that they practice.

The Transmission

गते गते पारगते पारसंगते बोधि स्वाहा ॥

gate gate pāragate pārasaṃgate bodhi svāhā

Far away and even further, passed and gone, I find myself.

—FROM *THE HEART SUTRA*

Many years ago in the early nineties, before there were yoga conferences, my teacher in India used to give what he called "yoga conferences," every day at five o'clock. Guruji would sit in his chair, his grandson Sharath sat in a smaller chair, and three or four of us would sit on the floor. In the morning, Guruji would say, "Today, five o'clock conference. You come." So we would all show up at five o'clock. When the clock hit 5:30, he'd say, "Thank you very much," and we'd leave.

Occasionally during the conference, a dog would come through the front door, and Guruji would shoo the dog away. Occasionally, a beggar would come and Guruji would send Sharath to get some money to give to the beggar. Occasionally, Guruji's wife would come in with cups of strong and sweet coffee. But most of the time those other things didn't happen and we just sat there for half an hour and then left.

When I attended these conferences, I would have a long walk back to where I was staying. There was a particular section of the walk that was crowded and congested, especially at that time of day—lots of taxis, buses, exhaust fumes, and people trying to sell you things or get something from you, or children wanting you to help them in some way. It was dense, noisy, and chaotic. After these conferences, when I walked through all that activity, I felt calm. I had awe for what was happening around me and I would think, "Wow! Life on the streets in India!" I had a kind of wonder about it all and people sort of picked up on it and would smile. Somehow in the half-hour that we sat with Guruji, even though he didn't tell us things, some kind of blessing was transmitted and it had its effect.

The Beautiful Alphabet

तदर्थ एव दृश्यस्यात्मा ॥ २१ ॥

tadartha eva dṛśyasyātmā

That which is seen is there to serve the seer.

—MASTER PATANJALI'S *YOGA SUTRAS*, BOOK TWO, SUTRA 21

Our world is made up of many different events, some good and some bad. All of it is there, however, to point out something. You don't have experiences just to say, "I've had so many experiences." Something is meant to unfold. That's what Master Patanjali is saying.

My husband's sister's little boy was turning three, and we wanted to get a present for him. Since we don't have children, we didn't know what to get the little boy. My husband asked some people whom he works with, and they told him we should get a train called the Thomas Train and that we could get it at the store Toys R Us.

On a very hot day in August, my husband said, "During my lunch break, I'm going to the Toys R Us to get the Thomas Train for Amadeo."

"You should sit down and eat lunch on your lunch break," I replied. "I'll go to the Toys R Us and get the Thomas Train."

"Fine," he said. So I went to the Toys R Us on 44th and Broadway in Manhattan to buy the Thomas Train. I had never been to the store before, but it was not what I was expecting. I was really quite unhappy in the store. Loud music was playing and it was extremely bright; mirrors were everywhere, and hordes of people. The shoppers were frantic, it seemed like they needed to get their toys quickly. It was intense.

I had just returned from India, where they love to serve, and I couldn't find anybody in Toys R Us who seemed to feel the same way. Finally, a very disgruntled worker told me the Thomas Trains were on the fifth floor. This upset me, because I knew I would want to get out of the store quickly, so to go to the fifth floor was getting myself deeper than I wanted to go into Toys R Us.

When I arrived on the fifth floor, I found the Thomas Train, which in my opinion was ugly. To me it had a kind of fast-food aesthetic. I asked someone why the train was so popular, and was told that it went with some DVDs. I didn't want to get the three-year-old Amadeo hooked on television, so I decided I didn't want to buy this train. I left the Toys R Us, and came home frustrated. I had spent the whole day on this train mission, but was empty-handed.

When my husband arrived home, I told him I hadn't bought the train and that I didn't like the scene in the Toys R Us or the train.

"Well, the boy's birthday is in two days," Robert said. "I'll go tomorrow during my lunch break."

"No," I responded. "I really think we should give something else to him. Don't worry about it, I'll think of something.

"Fine," he said.

The next day, I asked myself what gift for a three-year-old boy I would feel comfortable giving. I thought, "Well, he's three—just learning how to read. I could make a painting of the alphabet, with each letter a different color." Then I thought, "I'll put the Sanskrit alphabet on the back, so it will have two alphabets."

I took out my watercolors and made what I considered a nice gift. However, I didn't just sit down and draw that alphabet. There was a sequence of events and occurrences that led to a place where I was totally frustrated, and that made me think what else could I do; and then led me to create the gift that I felt was right.

Life is like that. It was an amazing sequence of events that brought me to my guru. Many people turn to a spiritual practice because of a sequence of events, and sometimes those events are quite dark. A sequence of events led me to my husband; somebody knew somebody who knew somebody. Anything creative that we do—writing a letter, cooking a meal, painting a picture—involves a sequence of events, a great deal of trial and error, and a lot of trying things this way and that.

In yoga, that sequence of events is considered holy and precious. We should examine and understand it, and we should not feel like a victim of the events in our life, but that there is some Divine order.

Meditation is incredibly helpful. If I had a better meditation practice, I would have known not to go to Toys R Us. I would have understood beforehand that I would not like the scene, not like the toy, and leave frustrated. If I had a better practice, I would have known not to go to all that trouble, and would have just sat down and painted the alphabet. Through meditation, you're able to see the sequence of events without actually going through it. This is what Master Patanjali is saying: the sequence of events can either just be a sequence of events, or you can recognize that the sequence has a purpose. It's not whether the sequences of events are good or bad: either can lead to the making of a beautiful alphabet.

Don't Divide the Fruit

The chanting of the holy scriptures had just ended. A Kashmiri lady brought a basket full of fruit, and offered it to Mataji. A little later, Mataji called two bhaktas [devotees] and asked them to distribute the contents of the basket.

"Give a whole fruit to each person," she said.

Someone who felt afraid that there might not be enough to go around objected. "Why a whole fruit? Would it not be safer to cut them into pieces?"

"No!" said Mataji. "Don't divide them. There is only one. All this is meant to make you grasp this. Whatever you do at any time no matter for what purpose must aim at the one. Then it will be complete. Indeed this holds good in every case. Everything is complete."

At this point, the lady who had brought the fruit suddenly got up and said, "When I was walking through the street carrying the basket, a cow followed me and tried to snatch some fruit. In spite of all my efforts to move the basket out of her way, the cow was so insistent that finally I gave her one of the fruits."

"Ah, that was my share," said Mataji. "It is complete."

—ANANDAMAYI MA

When I reflect on what Mataji said, I thought she would say, "Yes, divide the fruit and everyone will get their piece." When I was in India, every day at three o'clock I took Sanskrit classes that meant a lot to me. I had to go by rickshaw. There was one lady living nearby who also went to the class. So we decided to go together and share the rickshaw.

On the way, I would want to stop to buy flowers to bring to my teacher, and the lady I was with would never get any flowers. She'd sit in the rickshaw while I'd choose my flowers, and then we'd continue to class. Every day, I would offer the flowers to my teacher Jayashree, and she had none to offer. It bugged me that she never brought flowers, but I knew that I shouldn't judge her.

We rode together for a couple of months, and one day we got out of the rickshaw and walked toward the front door of Jayashree's house, when, without any thought at all, I turned and said to her, "Why don't you take these flowers and give them to Jayashree?"

She seemed to like that idea, and said, "OK. I'll do that."

"Great!" I said.

I gave her the flowers. We didn't divide the bouquet. I just gave them to her. We walked into the house. I had nothing. She had a beautiful bouquet. We went into the room and she said, "Jayashree, I'd like to give you these flowers."

Jayashree said, "Oh, they're so cute. I love yellow." I looked at my friend. She has blue eyes and they twinkled, and sunlight shone on her blond hair, and she looked perfect as she gave these flowers to the perfect teacher.

We are one body sharing one life. It doesn't matter who gives the flowers. By dividing everything, we reinforce our individuality. We can share without physically having our share.

Wanting Things and Not Wanting Things

अविद्यास्मितारागद्वेषाभिनिवेशाः क्लेशाः ॥ ३ ॥

avidyāsmitā rāga dveṣābhiniveśāḥ kleśāḥ

Absence of self-awareness, sense of ego, craving, hating, and fear of death are the mental afflictions that cause us pain.

—MASTER PATANJALI'S *YOGA SUTRAS*, BOOK TWO, SUTRA 3

Klesha means affliction, something that causes pain, an obstacle to happiness. Two of the five *kleshas* are *raga* and *dvesha*. *Raga* is craving—"I want that." *Dvesha* is aversion—"I don't want that." They are always put together, and said to be two sides of the same coin. Many commentaries on Patanjali's *Yoga Sutras* say that if a person doesn't have *raga*, they won't have *dvesha*.

Every summer I go to India with my dear friend Lisa to study yoga. Over the centuries, people have gone to India to buy exotic things. There are all kinds of textiles, such as carpets, shawls, and silks; jewels, such as gold, diamonds, and sapphires; oils, such as lemongrass, saffron, and jasmine; spices, such as cardamom, black pepper, and white pepper . . . so many things to buy.

We stay on the outskirts of town. There's not much to buy, only bananas and potatoes. I'm busy while I'm in India, but every now and then I have a free day from my classes, and of course I want to go to town. I'll say to Lisa, "Let's go shopping." She brings a list of things she wants to get: a bedspread made out of saris for her parents, a special robe for her writer friend, a thin white cotton blouse for her sister who lives in Phoenix where it's really hot, *The Brahma Sutras* in Sanskrit for her student, special herbs for her friend who's an Ayurvedic doctor. Her whole list is things she has thoughtfully picked out for other people.

Occasionally, there is something that she herself likes. She will say, "Oh! Look at that," and ask the merchant if she can see it. She'll ask how much it costs, but will never purchase it. I almost encourage her to buy it.

"Would you like it, Lisa?" I ask.

"No," she'll say. "I don't want it. I don't need it. It's nice, but what would I do with it?" It is like offering a plate of food to a person who's nauseous. Her lack of craving is admirable.

Dvesha is aversion. There are a lot of Westerners who get sick while in India. They come down with all kinds of ailments that one might have an aversion to, like boils, rashes, fevers, and terrible infections. Lisa, who is well trained in Ayurveda, gravitates toward people who become ill. One day, a fellow yoga student got a terrible rash, and immediately, I was afraid she might have touched me.

Lisa says, "I'm going to give her an oil rubdown with herbs," and off she goes with her bag of concoctions. This is how she lives her life, not craving and unafraid, and there's an air of heaven around her.

We want things and we don't want things. This is *raga/dvesha*. When we spend our energy in this way, we are bound to those things, and we're never satisfied. What's satisfying is our human decency and basic goodness, which are inside. Everything else only quenches our thirst temporarily. The deeper we go inside, the less we chase after things and run away from things outside. We lose interest, like the child loses interest in the toy after awhile.

Jayashree Has the Vedas

जितात्मनः प्रशान्तस्य परमात्मा समाहितः ।
शीतोष्णसुख दुःखेषु तथा मानापमानयोः ॥७ ॥

jitātmanaḥ praśāntasya paramātmā samāhitaḥ
śitoṣṇa-sukha-duḥkheṣu tathā mānāpamānayoḥ

The one who has conquered the mind, and reached the soul, is peaceful. To such a person, hot and cold, pleasure and pain, praise and blame are all the same.

—*THE BHAGAVAD GITA*, CHAPTER SIX, VERSE 7

My Sanskrit teacher lives in India. Besides being a Sanskrit scholar, she is an all-round scholar, and frequently gives lectures on different subjects. Often, she'll end our class early on account of a lecture she is giving. I'm always curious and ask, "Jayashree, what's the subject of your lecture tonight?" She says, "Astronomy, the stars," or, "Botany, the plants," or, "Medicine, herbs," or "Trigonometry, numbers," or, "Poetry, the arrangement of words," or, "Music, the embellishment of a note." These are all things she has said to me.

One time, I was admiring several paintings in her house, which I commented on, and she said, "Oh, I am making." She learned what she knows from books called the Vedas, which are said to be the oldest books in the world. She has them memorized.

She studied alongside her brother, who's actually her cousin, but she always calls him her brother. They studied these books together, late at night, once everyone had gone to bed. She wasn't encouraged to study these books. She was encouraged to do chores all day and into the night. By the time she had done all that was expected of her, it was bedtime. It was then that the two or them would burn the midnight oil studying these books. I never knew what this phrase "burning the midnight oil" meant until I pictured her and her brother doing exactly that, so they could see what they were reading. This is how she acquired her vast and deep knowledge, and became the head of the Sanskrit department of the university in Mysore.

Jayashree is married with children and grandchildren and lives with a large extended family. It seems to me that the relatives she lives with don't respect her or treat her nicely, and they're lazy. They're always sleeping on daybeds in the mainroom, watching TV, or reading the newspaper, while Jayashree is cooking, cleaning, sewing, studying, and teaching. I've always wondered about this situation.

One day, I showed up for class early as I always do, to get a spot next to Jayashree. She was in the kitchen washing heavy pots, the kind used to make rice for thirty people. Her relatives were lying on the beds. She was carrying a pot from the sink to the cupboard, and on her way she bumped into one of her relatives, who scolded her. "Look what you've done!" he said, pushing her. "You're getting fat, too." This upset me very much.

We went into the classroom, and Jayashree started getting the room ready for class, and I helped her. She was opening the windows, turning on the fans, laying out the straw mats, taking out the books, and she seemed totally unconcerned with what her relative had said.

"Doesn't it upset you when your relatives treat you like that?" I asked.

She turned to me. "What?" she said. She hadn't noticed what had happened. I was bringing it to her attention.

"Your relatives push you around and call you names. That doesn't upset you?"

She could see I was distraught, and she wanted to understand why. In order for her to understand, she had to travel down to my level. I could feel her traveling down, down, down. Then, again she said, "What?"

"Well, there was that thing with your relative and the pot. Didn't that upset you?"

And she said, "Oh, Ruth. You mustn't worry. It is not like that. I have the Vedas. I have knowledge. You mustn't worry. I have Sanskrit." If only I had that knowledge, then I wouldn't notice these things.

Meanwhile, her brother overheard and wanted to know what was going on. She told him, and he was chuckling. He thought it was so funny. The two of them were walking around chuckling. "We have Sanskrit. We have knowledge. We have the Vedas." I was amazed.

Most of us take things personally. If people are mean or criticize us, we take it personally. I know if somebody criticizes my work, I take it personally, because I've put so much love and care into it. This is OK. But, if we always take things personally, as a lifestyle, always having to defend and explain ourselves, it's a burden, and it's exhausting, and ultimately, it separates us from the knowledge.

I think that God has a plan, and if I'm busy justifying myself, I'll miss out on it.

Murata's Coat

A few years ago, I started seeing an acupuncturist, Kenji Murata. Sometimes he would ask, "What's new?" One time, I told him that, because I was unwell, I had stopped drinking black tea, and switched to green.

"Oh, you like green tea?" he said. "I have some." He went into his office, and came out with some green tea in a bamboo box that a patient of his had brought from Japan. "Take this green tea," he insisted.

Once, I told him that I had heard a piece of music by Edvard Grieg.

"Grieg, I have it!" he said. Then he played it during my treatment, and made me take the record home.

He was really hard to pay. If you gave him a check, he didn't cash it; he didn't take a credit card; and if you gave him cash, somehow when you got home the money was back in your pocket. He seemed to have no needs of his own and everything that others needed. I would go there with back pain and he'd spend the whole time on my ear.

I'd say, "Murata, it's my back."

He'd say, "Yes, I know," as he continued to put needles in my ear. I would leave and all of my back pain was gone. He had such knowledge of the body. I loved him very much.

At the same time, I had friend with cancer, named Asako. I arranged for her to see Murata. They were both Japanese, and they reminded me of each other. Murata was able to relieve some of her suffering and make her feel more comfortable.

Several months later, Murata passed away. It was very sad.

Later still, I met Asako in Tompkins Square Park in Manhattan. It was a very cold day, and she had on a wonderful coat. It looked warm, it was full length with a hood, and I was glad to see her wearing it. Because of her illness, she had become very thin and was cold all the time. Since she lived in California, she didn't have a lot of winter clothes, so I was impressed.

"What a beautiful coat," I said. "I am so happy to see that you're well-dressed on this cold day."

She said, "Yes, Murata gave me this coat. One day I went for a treatment and he thought I hadn't dressed warmly enough, and he insisted that I take it."

There he was, still answering to the needs of people, even after he'd passed away.

Some time passed, and Asako also died. I started to think about Murata's coat. I wondered where it was. I wanted it. The coat was a symbol of one person taking care of another. That is the purpose of life. And if you haven't realized that this is the purpose of life, to take care of others, that is ignorance."

The Lord Brings Rice

अपरिग्रहस्थैर्ये जन्मकथंतासंबोधः ॥ ३९ ॥

aparigraha sthairye janmakathamtā saṃbodhaḥ

When one does not grasp onto things, the reason for one's life, why one is born, and what is to become of them, becomes perfectly clear.

—MASTER PATANJALI'S *YOGA SUTRAS*, BOOK TWO, SUTRA 39

My friend Shakunthala volunteers in orphanages throughout the region where she lives. Everybody knows her, and the children love her. She's not afraid if a child is sick. She picks them up right away and gives them affection. I can't help worrying if the child's illness is contagious. It's great that there are people who aren't afraid. My husband's like that, too. He's a nurse. He just gets right in there. I'm a little more on the sidelines.

Shakunthala complains that the orphanages in India are all in the slums. "The slums are no place for a child to grow up," she says. She had the idea to have an orphanage in the countryside. The government of India sells land for noble causes at a cheaper price than other real estate. She applied for land. It took years, but the government accepted her application and is going to sell her a plot of land in the countryside. So I've been collecting money from many people to help her with this purchase. It's great, because if it were just my money, it wouldn't be as much.

I brought the money to the orphanage in the slums. They said they had been running low on rice, and then, "Now we will have a lifetime supply." They couldn't understand who I was, so they figured I was just the Lord Himself. That's how it is in India. They were so flabbergasted to have some strange Western woman just drop off a bundle of money, they didn't even thank me—they just kept thanking the Lord.

I felt grateful to be the messenger of the money, and to all of those who have faith in this project and care about the children over there.

Caring about others is what makes the world beautiful. If you are religious, then that quality of caring for others will keep the essence of your religion alive. If you're on a spiritual path, but you don't care about others, then, as my teacher would say, "You're not on a spiritual path. Only for thrills."

It's interesting that the more you care about others, the more your own needs decrease. You find that you're not buying the thing you already have. Instead, you're delivering money to an orphanage that is just about out of rice.

Corpse Pose

उत्तानं शववद्भूमौ शयनं तच्छवासनम् ।
शवासनं श्रान्तिहरं चित्तविश्रान्तिकारकम् ॥ ३४ ॥

uttānaṃ śavavad bhūmau śayanaṃ tacchavāsanam
śavāsanaṃ śrāntiharaṃ chittaviśrānti kārakam

Lying like a corpse with the mind and body dropped off,
completely at rest is savasana.

—*THE HATHA YOGA PRADIPIKA*, CHAPTER ONE, VERSE 34

This verse says that the yogi has the practice of playing with being dead—*savasana*. The world we live in is physical and material, and often the physical and material aspect of the world insists on being the only reality there is. We judge everything about our life and our success in that way—physically, materially.

Yoga teaches that there is a reality that exists beyond the physical and material one. We can call it the spiritual realm or the soul. When the mind and the body drop off, something continues. There is the expression "You can't take it with you to the grave" that addresses these different realities. What do you take with you to the grave? What can't you take with you? What lives on when the body and the mind drop off? The yogi has an interest in these questions, and through *savasana* we're able to practice this letting go of the material and physical world.

When my father passed away I reflected on whether there were signs of him letting go of the physical and the material world that maybe I didn't recognize. Because even though he was elderly when he died, I was surprised.

For the last fifteen years I'd gone out to California about four times a year to visit, more often over the last couple years, since my dad was getting so old. Each time, I would stay five or six days and on the evening before I left, my father would say to me, "Ruth, could you please come upstairs to my office?"

"OK," I would reply, and I would go upstairs to this little room, filled with books, scientific journals, ancient bank statements, and a big desk that was completely covered with papers.

"Sit down," he would say. "I want to reimburse you for your trip."

"Oh, that's not necessary, Dad," I'd respond.

"No, no," he'd insist. "I'll reimburse you."

Then he would pull out the drawer of the desk, and remove his checkbook, which was in a three-ring binder. He'd take out his nice old pen and put on his eyeglasses, and in his beautiful handwriting would write me a check for two hundred dollars.

"Now, go and put it in your wallet and then come back," he would say.

When I returned, he'd ask, "Did you put it in your wallet?"

"Yes, Dad, I did."

"That's good," he'd say.

It always seemed a little painful for him to go through this ritual with me. It wasn't that my father was stingy. He was thrifty, because he came to this country with ten dollars as a refugee at the age of eighteen. He had to take a train from New York City to Philadelphia, which meant that by the time he arrived he only had eight dollars left. He went from door to door selling silverware, which was of such poor quality that if you touched it too much it would get bent out of shape. As a young man, he suffered from starvation, tuberculosis, and typhoid, and as a result he was always frugal. He never stayed in fancy hotels or went to restaurants other than diners; and, if he'd had the opportunity, he never would have taken a taxi or spent four dollars on a fancy coffee.

In June, before I went to India, I visited my parents. Sure enough, on my last night there, my father asked me to come upstairs. He sat down at his table and wrote me a check for two thousand dollars.

"Dad," I said. "This is really not necessary."

"It's fine, it's fine," he replied. He didn't even say, "Put it in your wallet."

I thanked him, told him I could really use the money, and took it.

When I returned from India two months later, I visited my parents again, and at the end of the trip, my father said, "Come upstairs." Again, he wrote me out a check for two thousand dollars. It wasn't my birthday or a special occasion. When my husband visited by himself about eight weeks later, he told me on his return, "Your dad gave me three thousand dollars!"

At the time I thought, "Wow, it will be like this from now on!" But two weeks later, my father died, at the age of eighty-eight. As I reflected on these last generous gifts, I realized that my father was letting go—not only of his money, something material, but also of a strong personality trait in him, as well as his worries.

When we are facing death, if we're lucky enough to know it, it's a special time, a poignant time, and we have a clarity that allows us to do things that we might not normally do. In the practice of *savasana,* the yogi puts himself into a space that's poignant, that brings this clarity, so that we may actually do things that otherwise we would not.

Take Your Seat

सिद्धं पद्मं तथा सिंहं भद्रं चेति चतुष्टयम् ।
श्रेष्ठं तत्रापि च सुखे तिष्ठेत्सिद्धासने सदा ॥ ३६ ॥

siddhiṃ padmaṃ tathā siṃhaṃ bhadraṃ cheti chatuṣṭayam
śreṣṭhaṃ tatrāpi ca sukhe tiṣṭhet siddhāsane sadā

In the pose of perfection, lotus posture, lion posture, and gracious pose, always sit comfortably.

—*THE HATHA YOGA PRADIPIKA*, CHAPTER ONE, VERSE 36

When I brought my parents to see Guruji, my father was old and frail. Guruji, covered in ash and wearing nothing but a white cloth wrapped around his waist, was seated in a big, comfortable chair. Behind him was a window, and outside the window was the ocean. It was a fancy house that Tim Miller (one of the first Westerners to have received written permission to teach ashtanga yoga from Sri K. Pattabhi Jois back in the 1970s) had rented for Guruji, as he was teaching yoga for one week in Encinitas, in Southern California. This was the summer of 2005.

When we came in through the front door, Guruji stayed in his chair, but turned his head so he could see my father. Without getting up, he said with great warmth, "Come in. Come in," and waving his hand towards the grand collection of chairs, couches, and cushions, said, "Take your seat. Take your seat."

My father went and sat in the chair nearest the door, and my mother sat near Guruji. Guruji asked my father how old he was. Guruji told him that he looked very old, as if he had worked hard his whole life. He noticed my mother had an accent, and asked where she was from. She was happy to tell him, "Berlin, Germany." He asked her if she had grandchildren. She was also happy to tell him, "Two boys." Saraswati, Guruji's daughter, offered my parents some tea and dried fruits. My mother ate a date, and not knowing what to do with its pit, and realizing a holy family surrounded her, slipped the pit into her pocket. Sharath, Guruji's grandson, joined us briefly, just long enough to bow down to my parents. Sharath embodies humility.

Several days later my father said to me, "Your Guruji is an enlightened man." "Enlightened" is a word in my vocabulary, but not one I had ever heard either one of my parents use. I asked my father why he thought that, and he said because the first thing Guruji had said to him was, "Take your seat."

"Look at me, Ruth," my father said. "I can barely stand. You would think that people would offer me a chair if I'm left standing, but they don't. So I'm always afraid that I'll fall, and that's why I never leave the house. Had your Guruji gotten up, we would've had the introductions standing in the foyer. It would have been very difficult for me."

One of the last things my father said to me before he died was how much he enjoyed meeting Guruji. The word *asana* actually means "seat." The chair is the hieroglyphic of the Egyptian goddess Isis, the giver of life to all the creatures in the world, from the insect to the king.

In order to find our seat, we must offer a seat to others.

Being Together Is the Teaching

On his way from India to Florida, my Guruji spent a few days in New York City. One of my students arranged that I could stop by to see him. We were having coffee and chit chatting. There was no actual teaching going on. I asked Guruji what airline he'd come on. He said it was his own.

I said, "Your own airline, Guruji?"

He said, "Yes, no layover."

A wealthy student had arranged for him to fly on a private plane. Then Guruji told me who was on the plane: his daughter, his granddaughter, her husband, and two great-grandchildren. Then I asked him, "Did you take food on the plane?"

"Oh yes!" he said. His granddaughter had made food in Bangalore and they brought it with them on the plane.

He had been to the doctor that morning, so I asked him how his visit went. I told him that I wouldn't be in Florida for his classes, because I was leading a retreat that weekend. I said, "If I could be in two places at one time, I would definitely be there."

He said, "Oh, two places at one time? It is very difficult. Very difficult."

I noticed he had only one ring on. Usually he has a ring on every finger, and they're big and masculine. I asked, "Guruji, where are your rings?" He told me he'd forgotten them by the bath in Bangalore. Saraswati, his daughter, gave him her ring, because she said his hands looked so bare without any. So he was wearing this one woman's ring, and his hands looked beautiful.

Then another student came by to say "hi" to Guruji and she had a question for him. She asked, "Guruji, what is *Shivani Nadi*?"

Guruji said, "What?"

"*Shivani Nadi.* What is this? Isn't it near the naval?"

"Oh, *Shivani Nadi,*" Guruji responded. "I forgetting. I forgetting. I ninety-three years of my life finishing. Ninety-four starting. I forgetting." It was very sweet.

Then Guruji asked about my parents whom he had met and pointing his finger to his eye he said, "Your father—I looking, I looking your father." He remembered my father. They had met three years before. He forgot his rings, and he forgot what *Shivani Nadi* was, but he remembered my father.

We just had had this small talk, but his kindness came through in the small talk, and there wasn't any need for a teaching. It was just about being together. That was the teaching. Just being together. Not separate. Together.

You Pray God

On the morning of May 18, 2009, in his home, with his hand resting in his daughter's hand, and an upset stomach caused from an overload of medicine, Sri K. Pattabhi Jois passed away at the age of ninety-three, leaving the world with one less enlightened man.

For the last two years of his life, for the first time ever, he had been sick. He had grown thin, fragile, old. It surprised me to see him like this, because until he was ninety he was physically robust and powerful; whereas my father, with his bad circulation, his Ace bandages around his ankles, his pale skin, slow walk, and slumped-over posture, always was an old man to me. My love for Guruji as a frail man only increased. I worried whether he was uncomfortable, eating enough, if he had the right cane or not, or the right doctor. Caring for him in that way was the final blessing he gave to us all.

After his passing, there were days of prayers for the family members. On May 31, the last day of these prayers, the *puja* or service was open to anyone, and students from all over the world came, myself included. Everybody said the same thing: Any commitment that anyone had made for that weekend was "cancelable." We mirrored each other in our earnestness, and the local Indian people were impressed by our devotion. They said we had brought our hearts.

The *puja* itself was modest; it was in the Joises' home. There were flowers, but not so many. A few elderly men, very simply dressed, with low and quiet voices, did the singing. A pile of mail from around the world accumulated in the foyer and a few dogs hung around outside. Superficially, it didn't seem like much; essentially, it was perfect.

Early the next morning, the Bangalore airport was full of Guruji's students, going home to Hawaii, New York, Tokyo, London, San Francisco . . . all places. We shared stories with each other, and remembered what Guruji used to say before giving us physical adjustments.

"You pray God," he would yell.

And that was perfect, too.

About the Author

Ruth Lauer Manenti is the daughter of Lothar and Stefanie Lauer. Her parents came to the United States from Europe as refugees. Her father was a scientist and her mother is a published author. Ruth found her way to yoga twenty-five years ago after spending a year in bed due to a serious car accident. She has been teaching yoga for the past eighteen years to students from around the world, primarily at the Jivamukti Yoga School in New York City, her home. Ruth is a devoted student and has the blessings of her teachers: Sri K. Pattabhi Jois, Saraswati Jois, Sharath Rangaswami, Sharon Gannon and David Life, Dr. M. A. Jayashree, Prof. M. A. Narasimhan, Prof. Nagaraja Rao, and Dr. Gurudat and his family. Her husband, Robert, is a humble *tai chi* master and a gentle nurse who works with those in critical care at St. Vincent's Hospital in New York City. Ruth also has an MFA from the Yale School of Art, and sometimes teaches drawing and painting at Dartmouth College.

Donation

Because of the deep generosity that surrounds me, as well as the need we feel within our hearts to help others, a non-profit organization was set up in 2008 called Friends of Mysore Children. It was inspired by the Jois Charitable Trust, which was founded by Sri K. Pattabhi Jois to raise funds for those with extreme hardships, to protect the forests, and to encourage and maintain the ethical treatment of animals in India. As India has given us the teachings of yoga, it is only natural to give back.

Last year, Friends of Mysore Children gave a donation through the Jois Charitable Trust to the Chetana Trust, a small school that teaches special skills to people of all ages and backgrounds, whom society calls "disabled." The money we offered multiplied, because it was used to establish a program where the children make peanut, coconut, and cashew chocolates, shaped like sea shells and wrapped in colored foil, which many people buy.

If we contemplate what it means to a "slow learner," to be patiently and lovingly taught how to read or write, or how someone's life can change when they can create something and thereby bring home earnings, then it becomes impossible not to give at least something, if not everything.

One cannot forget when a child, holding a smaller child, pulls on your skirt out of hunger. That child is God, asking us to offer our best to the world.

A portion of the proceeds from this book will go to Friends of Mysore Children. If you would like to make an additional donation, please send to:

Friends of Mysore Children, Inc.
c/o Ruth Lauer Manenti
470 Stony Brook Road
Palenville, New York 12463

www.saraswatishands.org